Critical Care Medicine

Critical Care Medicine

Editor: Ronan Holland

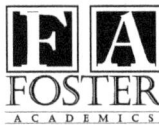

FA
FOSTER
ACADEMICS

www.fosteracademics.com

www.fosteracademics.com

FA FOSTER
ACADEMICS

Cataloging-in-Publication Data

Critical care medicine / edited by Ronan Holland.
       p. cm.
Includes bibliographical references and index.
ISBN 978-1-63242-640-6
1. Critical care medicine. 2. Emergency medicine. 3. Intensive care units.
I. Holland, Ronan.
RC86.7 .C75 2019
616.025--dc23

Foster Academics,
118-35 Queens Blvd., Suite 400,
Forest Hills, NY 11375, USA

ISBN 978-1-63242-640-6 (Hardback)

Contents

Preface VII

Chapter 1 **Current Status of Colonization and Infection by Multiresistant
Bacteria in the Spanish Intensive Care Unit: Resistance
Zero Program** 1
Miguel Ángel García García, Alfonso Martínez Cornejo,
David Arizo León and María Ángeles Rosero Arenas

Chapter 2 **Aneurysmal Subarachnoid Hemorrhage**..**24**
Adel E. Ahmed Ganaw, Abdulgafoor M. Tharayil,
Ali O. Mohamed Bel Khair, Saher Tahseen, Jazib Hassan,
Mohammad Faisal Abdullah Malmstrom
and Sohel Mohamed Gamal Ahmed

Chapter 3 **Current Perspectives on Cardiomyopathies** **51**
Nandita Mehta and Sayyidah Aasima tu Nisa Qazi

Chapter 4 **Severe Acute Pancreatitis and its Management**................................**72**
Arshad Chanda

Chapter 5 **Current Neonatal Applications of Point-of-Care Ultrasound** **94**
Jae H. Kim, Nikolai Shalygin and Azif Safarulla

Chapter 6 **Intensive Care Unit Workforce: Occupational Health and Safety** **109**
Melek Nihal Esin and Duygu Sezgin

Chapter 7 **Videolaryngoscopy in the Intensive Care Unit: We could Improve
ICU Patients Safety**..**127**
Eugenio Martínez Hurtado, Miriam Sánchez Merchante,
Sonia Martín Ventura, María Luisa Mariscal Flores
and Javier Ripollés Melchor

Chapter 8 **Abdominal Compartment Syndrome: What is New?**................................**173**
Abdulgafoor M. Tharayil, Adel Ganaw, Syed Abdulrahman,
Zia M. Awan and Sujith M. Prabhakaran

Permissions

List of Contributors

Index

Preface

This book has been a concerted effort by a group of academicians, researchers and scientists, who have contributed their research works for the realization of the book. This book has materialized in the wake of emerging advancements and innovations in this field. Therefore, the need of the hour was to compile all the required researches and disseminate the knowledge to a broad spectrum of people comprising of students, researchers and specialists of the field.

The branch of medicine concerned with the diagnosis and management of life-threatening conditions requiring sophisticated life support and monitoring is known as critical care medicine. Critical care is usually required to support unstable hypertension, acute renal failure, respiratory compromise, potentially lethal cardiac arrhythmias, or multiple organ failure. Intensive care is usually based upon a system-by-system approach to treatment. Gastro-intestinal tract, peripheries, cardiovascular system, endocrine system, hematology, microbiology, central nervous system, renal, and respiratory system are the nine key intensive care systems covered under the approach. All these nine key intensive care systems are considered on an observation-intervention-impression basis to produce a daily plan. This book unfolds the innovative aspects of critical care medicine which will be crucial for the progress of this field in the future. It elucidates new techniques and their applications in a multidisciplinary manner. As this field is emerging at a rapid pace, the contents of this book will help the readers understand the modern concepts and applications of the subject.

At the end of the preface, I would like to thank the authors for their brilliant chapters and the publisher for guiding us all-through the making of the book till its final stage. Also, I would like to thank my family for providing the support and encouragement throughout my academic career and research projects.

Editor

Current Status of Colonization and Infection by Multiresistant Bacteria in the Spanish Intensive Care Unit: Resistance Zero Program

Miguel Ángel García García,
Alfonso Martínez Cornejo, David Arizo León and
María Ángeles Rosero Arenas

Abstract

Current medicine, highly technified, and capable of amazing achievements, is not possible without the support of antibiotics. The problem of antibiotic resistance is almost as old as the antibiotics themselves. But at present, it is a serious threat to public health. We have to fight against antibiotic resistance in the hospital and in the out-of-hospital environment. The Resistance Zero program, promoted by the Spanish Society of Intensive Medicine, has achieved through a multidisciplinary approach with collaboration between doctors, nurses, cleaning staff and microbiologists, to control the colonization and infection by multiresistant germs in the environment of the Intensive Care Unit.

Keywords: antibiotic resistance, multiresistant bacteria, intensive care unit, colonization, infection

1. General concepts

1.1. Global data

The emergence of antibiotic and their use in clinical practice is one of the greatest achievements of Medicine. In the mid-twentieth century, its use became widespread, and it was thought that a rapid and definite eradication of infectious diseases was possible. However, the first resistant bacteria soon appeared, and antibiotic resistance has developed into a serious public health problem. It is estimated that up to 60% of nosocomial infections are caused by resistant germs both in Europe and in the United States. The Center for Disease Control and prevention (CDC) in the United States has estimated that the problem of antibiotic resistance is responsible for 2 million infections and 23,000 deaths per year with a direct cost of 20 billion dollars, and losses of productivity equivalent to 33 billion dollars [1]; the European Center for Disease Control, ECDC, have estimated that accounts for 25,000 deaths and 1.5 billion € per year by infections by multiresistant bacteria (MRB) [2]. Some consequences of this problem are: increased cost of health care, increased rates of failure of antibiotic treatment and increased mortality. This is not a problem limited to certain regions or countries and resistance can spread quickly in our globalized world.

1.2. Intensive care unit generalities

Intensive care unit (ICU) accounts for less than 10% of total beds in most hospitals, but more than 20% of nosocomial infections are acquired in ICU [3]. Acquired in ICU infections pose significant morbidity, mortality and expense; they are the most frequent cause of death in non-cardiac ICUs and 40% of all ICU expenses [4]. In comparison with patients from other areas of the hospital, ICU patients have higher chronic comorbidity, more severe acute physiological deterioration and are relatively immunosuppressed [5]. Its management also implies a high degree of invasiveness, with use of intravascular catheter, contact with a large number of health personnel—predisposing to colonization and infection—and are subjected to an increased colonization pressure [5].

When a patient goes to the hospital today, he undergoes a more effective and complete care than in previous years. Advances in diagnostic and therapeutic methods mean improvements in care and may be accompanied by a greater number of associated complications. All these data are magnified in ICU; ICU patients are more vulnerable to develop infections during their stay and to become colonized/infected with MRB. Overcrowding in closed areas of these severely ill patients with multiple comorbidities and subjected to invasive devices are risk factors for the development of nosocomial infections.

There is a clear relationship between the appearance of resistance and the highest antibiotic consumption. Infections due to resistant germs/MRB have limited therapeutic options, so inadequate empirical treatments are prescribed, the start of the correct treatment is delayed and therapeutic failures increase. All this leads to longer ICU stay, costs and mortality, with worse prognosis of the patient.

The highest density of MRB is observed in ICU. The importance of adequate and early treatment is greater in critically ill patients; for all above, it is necessary to implement programs for the prevention and treatment of multiresistant bacteria MRB, both in the ICU and in the community—a great number of MRB can be related to inadequate or excessively prolonged treatments in the general ward or outside the hospital.

1.3. Antibiotic resistance mechanisms

The mechanisms related to the emergence of resistance are varied. Resistance can be intrinsic or acquired. the first occurs in certain germs that are not innately sensitive to certain antibiotics, by a special membrane structure or related to the mechanism of the antibiotic. There may be at the molecular level: modifications in the targets (nucleic acid, ribosomes, action points of certain antibiotics—such as penicillin-binding proteins, PBPs); alterations in the transmembrane passage (porins, mechanisms of uptake or active transport); enzyme production (beta-lactamases). The appearance of mutations in the genetic material of the bacteria or the transfer of resistance genes from other germs explains the transformation from sensible to resistant bacteria. The exposure to antibiotics induces the disappearance of a population sensitive, and the selection of resistant strains to the antibiotics that end up being predominant.

1.4. Definition of MRB

MRB are defined as those microorganisms resistant to three or more antibiotics, which must also have clinical relevance. The exception to this rule is methicillin-resistant *Staphylococcus aureus* (MRSA) and vancomycin-resistant enterococcus (VRE) cases, in which the resistance condition is given by only one antibiotic. The phenomenon of resistance constitutes a medical problem, since it becomes a difficulty for the treatment and also epidemiological relevance, given the possibility of transmission of the outbreak. The ESKAPE (*Enterococcus faecium, Staphylococcus aureus, Klebsiella pneumoniae, Pseudomonas aeruginosa* and Enterobacter especies) are a specific group of bacteria with clinical relevance, associated with health care, and with the capacity to develop antibiotic resistance [6].

1.5. Description of the MRB

P. aeruginosa (Pa) has a predilection for humid environments and usually contaminates aqueous solutions such as disinfectants or soaps, mechanical ventilation equipment, fiberoptic bronchoscopes, and so on. Resistance may appear in the course of an antibiotic treatment. Its main mechanism of resistance is the presence of extended-spectrum beta-lactamases (ESBL) and alterations in permeability (porin mutations and expulsion pumps).

Acinetobacter baumannii (Ab) contaminates and endemically colonizes the hospital environment. It is capable of surviving and rapidly developing resistance to the main classes of antibiotics, more frequently in summer [7]. Some strains can survive to environmental drying form months, which facilitates transmission via contamination of fómites in the hospital. The health personnel is usually carrier of Gram-negative bacilli (GNB) (30%). Outbreaks have been described in relation to contaminated mechanical ventilation equipment and manual transmission. Infections have also been described in war wounds and in situations of natural disasters. Sixty-three percent of bacterial isolation from war wounds in Iraq and Afghanistan corresponded to this germ [8]. Infections tend to appear in patients with long stay in the ICU and health centers, dependent on mechanical ventilation, central catheter carriers, and with prior treatment with third-generation cephalosporins, fluorquinolones or carbapenemes. Although patients with Ab infection have high mortality, it is not clear whether mortality can be attributed to infection or to life-threatening conditions [9]. Several factors are associated with mortality: isolation in blood cultures, presence of signs of sepsis/septic shock, resistance to imipenem, longer stay in ICU, pneumonia and diabetes mellitus [10]. Cases of community acquisition have been described in situations of chronic obstructive pulmonary disease (COPD), diabetes, alcoholism and cancer [11]. It has great capacity to acquire and accumulate resistance genes from other GNB via plasmids/transposons, with low permeability for many antibiotics, constitutive ejection pumps, production of beta-lactamases and so on.

Klebsiella pneumoniae (Kp) contaminates the medical material although its main reservoir is the digestive tract and the hands of the health care personnel from where it can give rise to epidemic outbreaks. Its main mechanism of resistance is the production of beta-lactamases. The genes that encode them are transmitted by plasmids, which contribute to their rapid diffusion among other GNB.

MRSA shows resistance to methicillin by means of a protein encoded in the mecA gene and transported in the chromosomal cassette SCCmec. The frequent use of vancomycin has led to the emergence of strains with intermediate or complete resistance to vancomycin by acquisition of the gene through a plasmid. They currently constitute up to 50% of Staphylococcus infections.

1.6. Factors that predispose to infections by MRB

Certain elements as advanced age, functional dependence, cognitive deterioration and comorbidities, prolonged hospital stays, contact with personnel sanitary, intravascular catheters, bladder catheterization, previous antibiotic treatment, and so on, contribute to an increased selective pressure (leading to the emergence of MRB) and increased colonization pressure (through an ineffective environmental containment) [11].

1.7. Consequences of infection by MRB

The prognosis of MRB infections is not good, with an increase in hospital stay, mortality and economic costs [12]. These types of infections are usually resistant to empirical therapies, which implies a delay in starting the correct antibiotic treatment. Also derived from this, the use of second line treatment with lower bactericidal capacity and less favorable pharmodynamic/pharmacokinetic profile contributes to a higher incidence of adverse events. At times, a greater virulence of these germs has been described.

1.8. Colonization and infection

The difference between these two terms lies in the simple presence (colonization) or clinical involvement (infection). The oropharynx is colonized early by hospital flora, especially GNB, in critically ill patients. The risk of colonization increases with hospital stay and severity. In the same way, the administration of antibiotics systemically increases the risk of acquiring the carrier state. Patients with APACHE II greater than 20 are usually carriers of abnormal flora such as GNB and MRSA. The passage from colonization to infective germs is defined by the rupture of the natural defense mechanisms (neutropenia, immunosuppression), the pathogenicity of the germ itself, alteration of the intestinal flora by antibiotic therapy previously administered. Altered mechanisms of clearance of germs are suggested. A necessary factor for the development of the infection is the overgrowth; 20–40% of carrier patients develop an infection, so those carriers must be actively identified when we want to control an outbreak of infection by resistant flora.

1.9. Exogenous-endogenous infections in the ICU

Infections can be classified according to origin and carrier status:

- Exogenous: nonpreceded by digestive colonization. The infective flora is endemic to the ICU. It constitutes 10–15% of the infections acquired in critical care.

- Endogenous: preceded by colonization of the digestive system by potentially pathogenic germs (PPG). It is endogenous primary if the patient already has them at the time of admission. It is usually precocious and represents 50% of registered infections. The endogenous secondary is caused by germs acquired in the ICU and colonizes the patient before causing the infection. They represent 35–40% of infections acquired in critical care.

The multimodal prevention of nosocomial pneumonia is based on these concepts. Primary endogenous pneumonias can be prevented with a short course of antibiotics such as cefotaxima that eliminates the colonizing germs of the oropharynx and upper respiratory tract of the carriers. Endogenous pneumonia is treated with the prevention of the carrier state with enteral antibiotics (PPG will not be able to adhere the coated mucosa of antibiotics). Exogenous pneumonia is prevented with hygienic measures.

1.10. Mechanisms of appearance and extension of resistance

The main responsible for the emergence and extension of resistance are the indiscriminate use of antibiotics and the transmission of resistant microorganism between humans (or between human and environment). The antibiotics exert a selective ecological pressure on the bacteria, thus promoting the appearance of resistance germs. Inadequate practices of prevention of the infection along with inadequate hygienic measures will favor the extension of the bacteria. The strategies to avoid these phenomena are aimed at a better use of antibiotics (reducing the selective pressure) and optimizing the infection control measures (reducing the colonization pressure) [13, 14].

Some measures aimed at a rational use of antibiotics are the following:

- Evaluation committees: formed by clinicians, pharmacists and microbiologists; pursue the effective and safe use of antimicrobials, evaluate and guide decision making; and implement educational programs to improve the use of antibiotics;

- implementation of clinical guidelines and protocols to promote the proper use of antibiotics;

- to use a form with pre-authorization for broad-spectrum antibiotics (non-specific restriction);

- preferred use of limited spectrum antibiotics (first-generation cephalosporin);

- personalized audit (mandatory consultation with infectious disease specialists to improve the appropriateness of antibiotic therapy and to reduce the use of broad spectrum antibiotics);

- to use predictive scores for MRB infections can be useful to minimize both the time to initiate appropriate antibiotic treatment and the unnecessary use of broad spectrum antibiotics.

While some measures of patient-patient transmission control are:

- hand washing;

- contact isolation measures (very important in case of MRSA, ERV and germs producers of ESBL), even grouping the colonized/infected patients (cohorting) and having staff exclusively dedicated to the care of these infectious patients;

- the use of universal contact precautions is not clear in all patients admitted to ICU;

- cutaneous decolonization/daily bath with chlorhexidine to colonized/infected patients (despite the limitations of the current studies) [15];

- decolonization of the upper respiratory tract and gastrointestinal tract. Several options: oropharyngeal decontamination with antiseptics (chlorhexidine); selective oropharyngeal decontamination (with nonabsorbable antibiotics applied to the oropharynx); and selective digestive decontamination (with nonabsorbable antibiotics applied to the oropharynx with intravenous antibiotics);

- surveillance of early infections by MRB (for early identification of these germs, control of outbreaks—imited in time—and situations of endemic increase of isolation);

- to implement strategies of infection prevention in relation to invasive devices (reduce the use of central venous catheters, bladder catheters, orotracheal tubes, etc);

- to regulate and monitor the process of cleaning, disinfection and environmental sterilization.

1.11. Proper antibiotic treatment

The evolution of an infectious process depends on the characteristics of the initial focus, the hemodynamic parameters, host factors, the responsible pathogen, in vitro antibiotic susceptibility tests and the precocity of the appropriate antibiotic treatment. The use of antibiotics is, at the same time, part of the problem and the solution when we talk about antibiotic resistance. Unfortunately, the emergence of resistance is faster than the creation of new antibiotics by the pharmaceutical industry. In general, the solution involves a global reduction in the consumption of antibiotics, although it is necessary to implement control programs aimed at rationalizing their use.

A frequently forgotten fact is that the majority of antibiotic consumption is done at the extra-hospital level (Primary Care and food industry) [16]; it is necessary to regulate its use. Up to 50% of antibiotics prescribed at the hospital level are unnecessary, many of them are broad spectrum. The inadequate use of antibiotics increases the mortality of patients with severe sepsis, subjects them to unnecessary adverse effects and generates unjustified expenses. On the other hand, it is of vital importance to define the role of prophylactic antibiotic treatment and also differentiate the systemic inflammatory response syndrome of any cause from a real infectious process.

The loss of sensitivity to antibiotics is to be solved with several strategies: to speed up the development of new antimicrobials—the initiative "10 × 20" of the IDSA; 10 new antimicrobians available on 2020; to improve the mechanisms of infection control in health centers; and to optimize the use of current antibiotics with the intention of extending their useful life. An adequate administration of antibiotics should be based on the following principles:

- early start (associated with microbiological cultures);

- proper choice of antibiotic: based on local ecology and habitual patterns of resistance;

- suitable doses, based on pharmacokinetic and pharmacodynamics data, taking into account that in critical patients the increase in volume of distribution, cardiac output and glomerular filtration requires the administration of doses that could be above the usual doses (currently available antibiotics rarely cause serious adverse effects);

- evaluate the need to maintain the started treatment: to remove unnecessary antibiotics by culture results, and if possible, to narrow the spectrum (de-escalation);

- adequate duration of antimicrobial treatment (usually too long due to the absence of evidence of optimal duration and for fear of suspending it if the evolution of the patient is good).

Different strategies have been described and tested to avoid resistance to antibiotic. Rotation consists of restricting in an established way an antibiotic or a class of antibiotics during a certain period of time, to reintroduce it later; the aim is to reduce the selective pressure exerted on the microbial flora and to minimize the appearance of resistance to rotated antibiotics. Cycling is to prescribe antibiotics according to a pre-established a priori sequence. In scheduling, an antibiotic or antibiotic class is replaced by another antibiotic or class with a comparable antimicrobial spectrum; there is change to another antimicrobial without returning to the initial agent. In rotation, there is a circular pattern. The usefulness of these strategies is theoretical. Periodic modifications would limit the generation of resistances by avoiding prolonged exposures to the same antimicrobial agent; the restriction of an antibiotic can result in the compensatory potentiation of the use of other unrestrained agents, with a later increase of resistance to these second agents. Also, the elimination for the selective pressure by an antibiotic when withdrawing its use does not imply the eradication of the genetic material responsible of the resistance. Despite the theoretical benefits of these strategies, their results are contradictory, and none of them have showed real benefit so far [17].

1.12. Epidemiological surveillance: multimodal prevention program

Epidemiological surveillance consists of the systematic collection, analysis and interpretation of data about a problem related to public health. The implementation of multimodal prevention programs must have the following elements: identification of problems, implementation plan, involvement of managers, record of compliance with objectives and, finally, the analysis of obstacles that may arise. An essential aspect of these programs is learning: the absence of adherence to the measures of the program due to lack of information or insufficient learning time should be avoided.

The antimicrobial stewardship programs bring together specialists in infectious diseases, clinical pharmacologists, clinical microbiologists, epidemiologists and other, sometimes also intensivists, all of them gathered for the purpose of an adequate prescription of antibiotics. But this is just one aspect of a complex problem like antibiotic resistance.

The 12 steps described by the CDC to prevent antibiotic resistance are the following:

- prevention of the infection:
- vaccine administration;
- removal the catheters (as soon as possible);
- effective diagnosis and treatment of the infection:
- analyze the sensitivity of the germ and to adapt the treatment to the pathogen;
- discuss with experts;
- appropriate use of antimicrobials:
- antibiotic control;
- knowledge of local microbiological data;
- treat the infection, not the colonization or the contamination;
- know how to refuse vancomycin;
- stop antibiotic treatment if patient has healed (propose the reduction of antibiotic treatment according to the clinical situation of the patient);
- prevention of the transmission:
- isolate the pathogen;
- break the chain of infection.

2. Resistance Zero (RZ) project

The Spanish Society of Intensive Care (SEMICYUC) has developed several projects with the aim of reducing infectious events (nosocomial infections): Bacteremia Zero (BZ) (catheter-related bacteremia) and Pneumonia Zero (NZ) (pneumonia associated with mechanical ventilation). After the implementation of these projects, a sustained decrease in the rate of such infections, and globally nosocomial infections has been achieved (**Figure 1**). It has been described that, surprisingly, the rate of pneumonia associated with mechanical ventilation began to decrease with the start of the BZ Project.

The last project carried out is Resistance Zero (RZ). Its objectives are:

- Primary: reduce by 20% the appearance of one or more MRBs of Nosocomial origin that are identified during their admission in ICU;

- Secondary: describe the MRB map in spanish ICUs, differentiating those identified at the time of admission to the ICU and those that appear after 48 h of stay; promote and reinforce the safety culture in them; and create a network of UCIs, through the autonomous communities, that apply safe practices of demonstrated effectiveness.

The aim of the project is to minimize the three factors that influence the appearance of MRB in critical patients: the adequate prescription of antibiotics, the early detection of MRB and

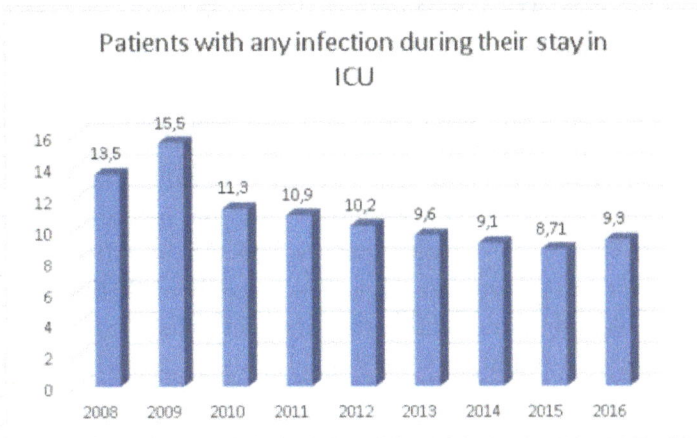

Figure 1. Decrease of acquired in ICU infection rate (patients with acquired in ICU infections for every 100 patients admitted to the ICU) during the different zero projects. Start of BZ 2009: Start of NZ 2011; start of Resistance Zero 2014.

the prevention of its spread/cross colonization, and the elimination of reservoirs. The MRBs in follow-up are: MRSA, VRE, Enterobacteria resistant to third generation cephalosporins, especially the ESBL producers, and those resistant to carbapenems, especially the carbapenemase producers; *P. aeruginosa* resistant to> = 3 families of antibiotics including: carbapenems, cephalosporins, piperaziline/tazobactam, fluoroquinolones, aminoglycosides, colistin; and *Acinetobacter baumannii* resistant to carbapenems.

The recommendations of the project are:

1. Identify in each ICU at least one intensivist physician responsible for the control of antibiotics, with experience in surveillance and infection control and in the management of antibiotics. Systematically evaluate the use of antibiotics in ICUs and advise physicians responsible for patients with the intention of assessing reasons for prescription (indication), assessing choice and correct administration (dose, interval, duration) and possibility of withdrawal or adjustment.

2. Administer antibiotics empirically active against MRB only in infections with systemic response (severe sepsis, septic shock (SS)), and high suspicion of being MRB based on present risk factors and local epidemiology. In other cases, it is recommended to use lower spectrum antibiotics and/or wait for microbiology results to start antibiotics directed to MRB (carbapenems, colistin, tigecycline, glycopeptides, daptomycin, linezolid). In critical surgical patients with infection data but without sepsis/SS, the start of antibiotic treatment can be delayed until microbiological confirmation, without this implying an increase in mortality or stay in the ICU.

3. Designate a nurse as a project reference and responsible for the control of precautions directed to preventing the transmission of MRB. Ensure the effective implementation of the handwashing strategy, and dispose of an alcohol-based preparation dispenser in each bed.

4. Perform an active search for the presence of MRB in all patients at the time of admission to the ICU, and at least once a week throughout their stay. The type and number of samples will be chosen according to the local epidemiology, and at a minimum, they will include

nasal, rectal and oropharyngeal swabs (tracheal aspirate in intubated patients); in addition, you can take other samples to control possible reservoirs (infections, skin ulcers, etc.). The samples will be processed to identify the MRBs recommended by the local epidemiology, according to Microbiology and the infection control teams of each hospital.

5. At the time of admission of each patient in ICU, a checklist that includes several items (hospital admission>5 days in the previous 3 months, institutionalized-prison, social health centers, nursing homes-, colonized or infected by MRB) will be completed., antibiotics> = 7 days in the previous month -especially with third and fourth generation cephalosoporins, quinolones and carbapenemics-, chronic renal failure undergoing hemodialysis or chronic ambulatory peritoneal dialysis, and chronic pathology with a high incidence of MRB colonization/infection-cystic fibrosis, bronchiectasis, chronic ulcers-) with the objective of identifying those patients with high risk of being carriers of MRB. In patients with one or more risk factors, preventive contact precautions will be applied, and surveillance culture samples will be collected.

6. Control compliance with the different types of precautions that should be applied: standard, or based on transmission mechanisms (isolation). The precautions will vary according to the identified MRB and its transmission mechanism (drops, air, and contact). They are mandatory standards for all health personnel and for the families of the patient. Nursing empowerment must be recognized to control strict compliance. The presence of necessary material for its application must also be facilitated. Contact isolation should be practiced with the use of a coat and gloves before contacting the patient, and removing them before leaving the patient's environment (for a single use).

7. Have an updated protocol for daily and terminal cleaning of rooms occupied by patients with MRB. Several aspects must be agreed with the cleaning and Preventive Medicine teams of the hospital: the cleaning method (method, frequency, products, etc.) according to the type of surface and the fixed structures present, including the beds.

8. Elaborate a document for cleaning the clinical material and scanning devices in the ICU, commonly used in hospitalized patients, assessing whether cleaning, disinfection or sterilization is necessary. The importance of cleaning the sanitary material (fondendoscopes, fiberoptic bronchoscopes, etc.) and nonsanitary (computer keyboards, landline and mobile phones, keys, etc.) usually used in the ICU should be made aware. It is the responsibility of each worker to clean and disinfect appliances for personal use.

9. Include products containing chlorhexidine (4% soaps or other products impregnated with 2%) in the daily hygiene of patients colonized/infected with MRB, in addition to the obvious need for cleaning to eliminate organic waste.

10. Given the suspicion of an epidemic outbreak, it is recommended to typify at a molecular level the causative microorganism to know the clone responsible for the outbreak and its traceability. Studies of outbreaks based on phenotypic characteristics (antigenic, metabolic or antibiotic resistance properties) are insufficient to establish conclusive differences or similarities between microorganisms. The molecular typing allows us to know the transmission mechanisms of the pathogen to establish measures that prevent its dissemination. The centers that do not have means can submit the microbiological samples to the Resistance Vigilance Program of the National Microbiology Center of the Carlos III Health Institute (Madrid).

As additional recommendations, hand hygiene is very important, with the use of hydroalcoholic solution by health personnel before and after patient care. It is the most effective measure for the transmission of germs. Its purpose is to prevent the transmission of microorganisms in a bidirectional way between professionals and patients, besides protecting the care environment of pathogenic microorganisms. The priority method to perform hand hygiene in the absence of organic matter or visible dirt is the friction with alcohol-based products. They will not be used in case of contact with patients/surfaces contaminated with spores (C difficile). Gloves should be worn in several situations: when handling blood or body fluids, mucous membranes or non-intact skin, when transporting or touching surfaces stained with blood, liquids or body fluids, or performing any procedure of blood extraction or parenteral treatment. They must be changed if they are broken or contaminated, between one patient and another, and between procedures in the same patient. The misuse of gloves increases the risk of pathogen transmission, and its use never substitutes for hand hygiene.

The indicators used in the RZ project are:

- Rates of patients with one or more BMR acquired in ICU: number of patients admitted to the ICU with 1 or more MRBs identified after 48 h of admission (and up to 48 h after discharge from the ICU) for 1000 days of stay in ICU, or by 100 patients admitted. MRBs are evaluated in clinical samples (infections or colonizations) and in surveillance samples, but not in environmental samples.

- Rate of days free of antibiotics: number of days—patient who does not receive systemic antibiotics for 1000 days of ICU stay. All systemic antibiotics are included regardless of the reason for their use.

- Rate of antibiotic use in infections acquired in ICU: number of days - patient with systemic antibiotic treatment for infections acquired in ICU, for 1000 days of ICU stay.

The project is complex and flexible, and adapts to the reality of each hospital. It is also contemplated to apply an integral security plan that seeks to promote and strengthen the safety culture in the daily work in the ICUs. Health professionals who provide critical care to the critically ill patients must be aware of the security risks of our units. The culture in general safety of the unit must be evaluated. We must work proactively on the potential risks of critical patient care, and propose recommendations based on daily practice that tries to minimize them. The notification of errors should be encouraged, and a goal of improvement should be proposed over time, with follow-up of proposed measures to achieve it. We have developed daily checklist tools that assess the safety of the patient on a daily basis in the different spheres of their management, and even a list of daily objectives—need of tubes/catheters, assessing whether parenteral medication can be suspended or passed to oral route, possibility of discharge from the ICU, and so on.

This project has preceded and promoted the creation of a new National System for the Surveillance of Infection Related to Health Care in Spain, in agreement with the Ministry of Health.

3. European data. ECDC

Data on infections associated with healthcare acquired in ICU are assessed by the ECDC. Recent data (2015) [1, 2] show that 8.3% of patients who remain in the ICU for more than

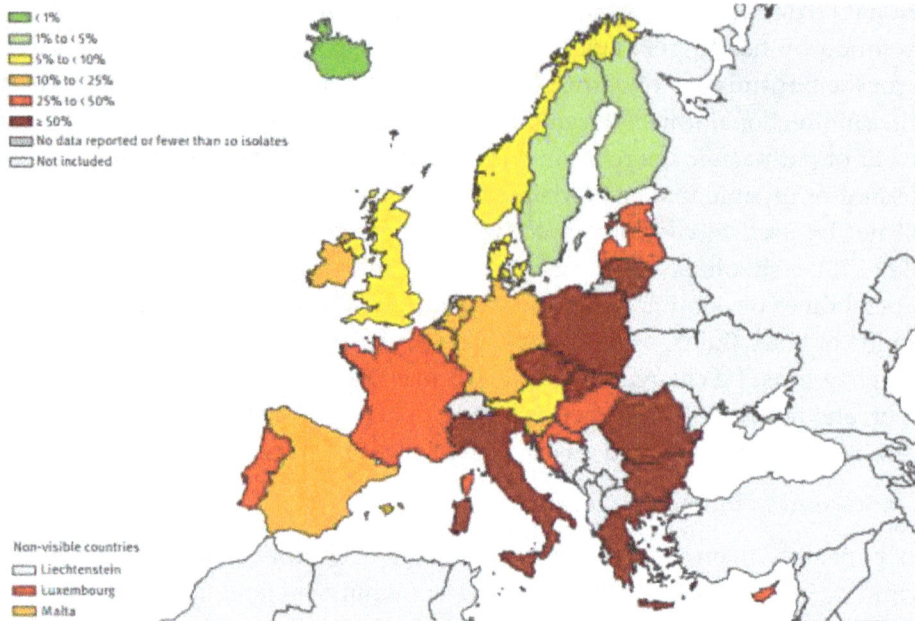

Figure 2. North-south and west-east gradient of % resistance of *K. pneumoniae* to third generation cephalosporins.

48 h develop at least one infection (pneumonia, bacteremia or urinary tract infection). The most frequent causal germs are *P. aeruginosa* (pneumonia), *Staphylococcus* spp. coagulase-negative (bacteremia) and *Escherichia coli* (urinary tract infections). On average, 23.1% of *S. aureus* are MRSA; 3.4% of Enterococci are VRE. Resistance to third generation penicillin is described in variable percentages in E coli (20%), Klebsiella (43%) and Enterobacter (42%); resistance to carbapenems is also noticeable in Klebsiella (11%), *Pseudomonas aeruginosa* (24%) and *Acinetobacter baumannii* (69% of averages). In a report of the European Antimicrobial Resistance Surveillance Network (EARS-Net) of 2016 [2], the main surveillance system in the European Union on bacteria that can cause serious infections, broad variations are described in relation to bacterial species, antimicrobial group and geographical region. For many combinations of bacterial species (*E. coli, K. pneumoniae, P. aeruginosa, Acinetobacter, S. aureus, Enterococcus*)—resistance to antimicrobial groups, there is a growing gradient from north to south, and from west to east, perhaps in relation to variations in the use of antimicrobials, infection prevention and control practices, and differences in diagnosis and healthcare utilization patterns between countries [18]. Overall, there seems to be a slowly increasing resistance over time (in the 2013–2016 interval) of E coli resistant to one of the three key antimicrobial groups (fluoroquinolones, third generation cephalosporins and aminoglycosides), with a tendency to stabilize the percentage of *K. pneumoniae* resistances (**Figure 2**).

4. Global data in Spain: ENVIN study: RZ project

The national study of nosocomial infection surveillance (ENVIN) represents the effort maintained over time (since 1994) to know and reduce the prevalence of nosocomial infection in ICUs. It describes nosocomial infections (NI) acquired in ICUs associated with invasive instrumentation. The data are collected mainly during the second quarter of the year (few units carry out the project throughout the year). The more frequent NI in the ICU are urinary infections associated with urinary catheter (31.87%), followed by ventilation-associated pneumonia (29.97%) and bacteremia (catheter-associated bacteriemia in 11.31%). In recent years, there has been a relative increase in the former ones and a decrease in the latter. The most frequently isolated germs in ICU infections (excluding bacteremia from other foci) are: *E. coli* (14.1%), *P. aeruginosa* (12.9%), *K. pneumoniae* (9.8%), *S. epidermidis* (8.2%), *S. aureus* (4.9%), *C. albicans* (4.8%), *E. cloacae* (3.5%), *S. marcescens* (2.7%), and so on. The type of reported patients is variable: medical (44%), 19.5% of surgeries scheduled, 10.3% of urgent surgeries and 19.8% of coronary patients. The extrinsic risk factors for nosocomial infections are: antibiotics before admission (21.1%), antibiotic treatment in ICU (64%), surgery in 30 days before (32.8%), urgent surgery during their stay in ICU (10.2%), central venous catheter (63.9%), mechanical ventilation (42.4%), bladder catheter (76.4%), parenteral nutrition (8.3%), and so on.

The implementation of the RZ project is more complex than the previous programs. It involves the collaboration of more staff and services, so the number of participating ICUs has been lower (of>190 in the first two projects, compared to 103 in RZ). In the following graphs, the evolution of the different indicators collected in the project is reviewed.

The evolution by quarters of the frequency of colonization/infection of patients with MRB, per 100 patients admitted, throughout the development of the RZ project is observed in **Figure 3**, with an ascending tendency with peaks coinciding with the collection periods of data from the ENVIN project (second quarter of each year). The average value throughout the project is 6.23 patients per 100 admissions. The colonization/infection plot for 1000 stays is similar.

Throughout the RZ project, there is an increase in the isolation of germs at the admission (acquisition prior to admission to the ICU) versus isolation during their stay (discrete decrease),

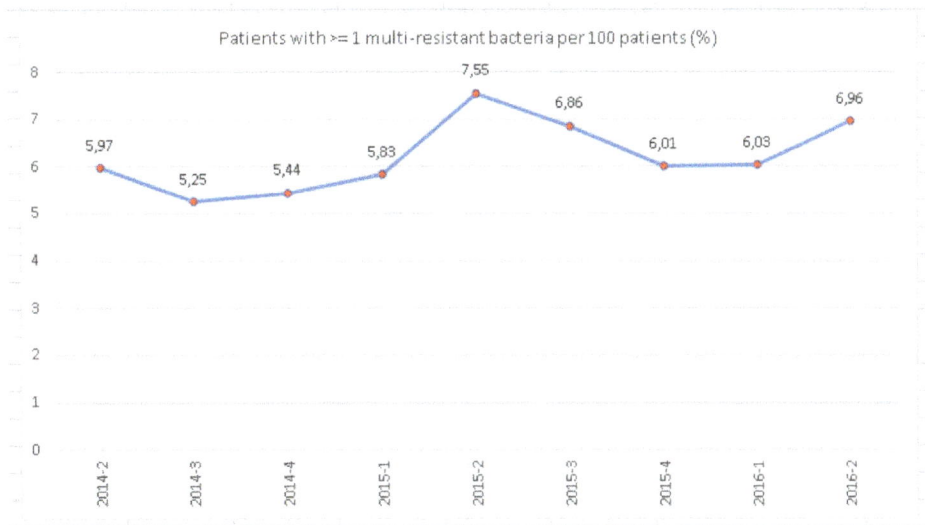

Figure 3. Temporal variation of the rate of MRB colonization/infection in ICU.

taking into account colonizations and infections (**Figure 4**). The average value during the project is 3.84 patients% (previous) and 2.60% (during), with an increase of the previous ones of 26% and a decrease of those acquired during the ICU admission of 16.7%.

In relation to the germs acquired in the ICU, there was a slight increase in colonization (5%) and a significant decrease in MRB infections (45%) (**Figure 5**), with average values of 1.75% patients colonized and 1.09% of infected.

Figure 1 (see above) and the following ones (**Figures 6–8**) show the tendencies initiated with the BZ and NZ projects of descent of patients admitted to the ICU with an infection (up to 8.7%, **Figure 1**), of reducing the use of antibiotics (up to 19.5% of patients, **Figure 6**), of reducing the days of antibiotic treatment (DOT, up to 109.7 per 1000 stays, **Figure 7**) and increasing days without antibiotic treatment (up to 40%, **Figure 8**). A rate of 2.15 antibiotics per patient with antibiotic treatment is described in 2016.

MRB colonization-infection rates change in successive years (**Figure 9**), with significant increases in enterobacteria carrying ESBL and carbapenemases and decrease in *A. baumannii*, *P. aeruginosa* and MRSA.

We can distinguish between the isolation of germs upon admission and during their stay, which can allow us to distinguish the predominant MRB germs that the patient "brings" to the ICU with those that he/she "acquires" during his stay. **Figure 10** shows that Acinetobacter infections appear mostly during their stay, against infections by ESBL-producing germs that are mostly present at admission.

Figures 11 and **12** show an important variability in the different autonomous communities, both in the MRB isolation rate (global of 6.23 per 100 patients) and in the isolated MRB types, for a total of 3195 isolated MRBs.

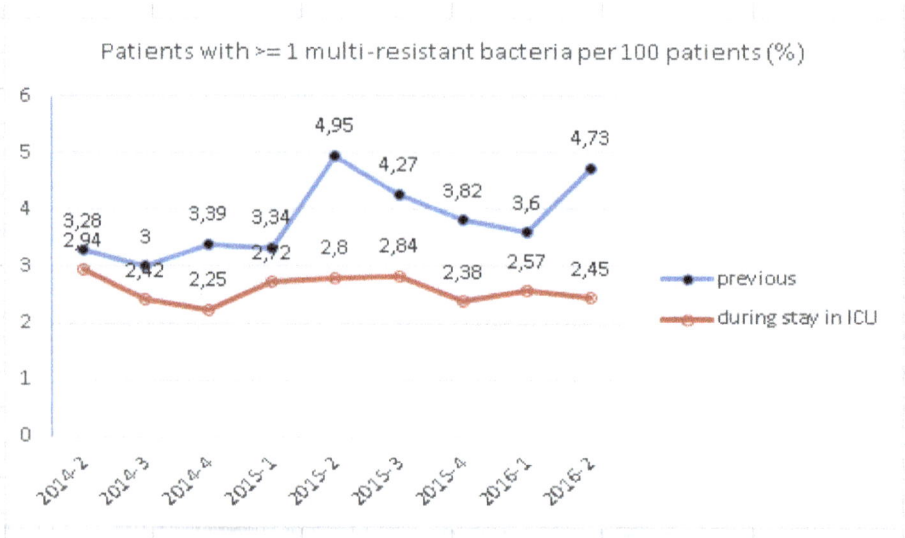

Figure 4. Evolution of BMR isolates prior to admission to the ICU and during admission.

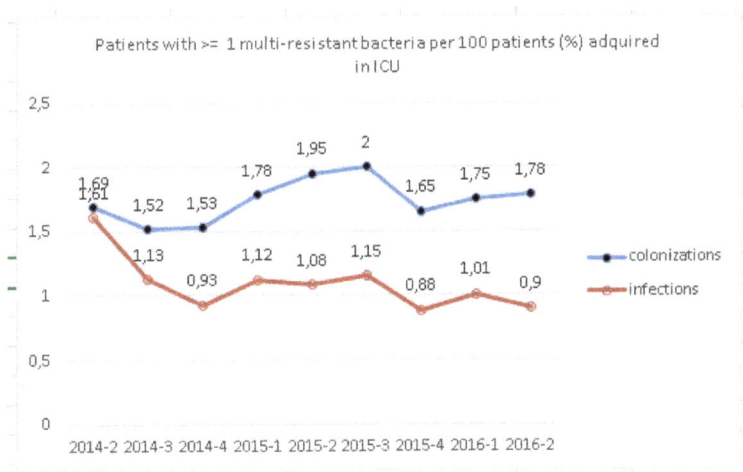

Figure 5. Evolution of colonized and infected patients during their stay in the ICU.

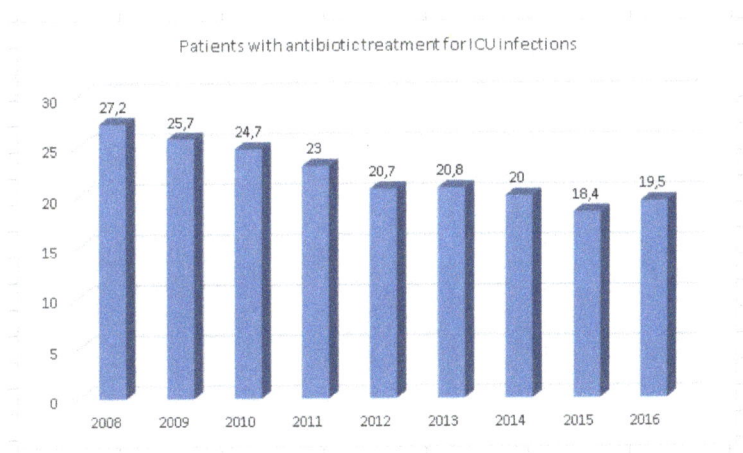

Figure 6. Reduction in the use of antibiotics over time.

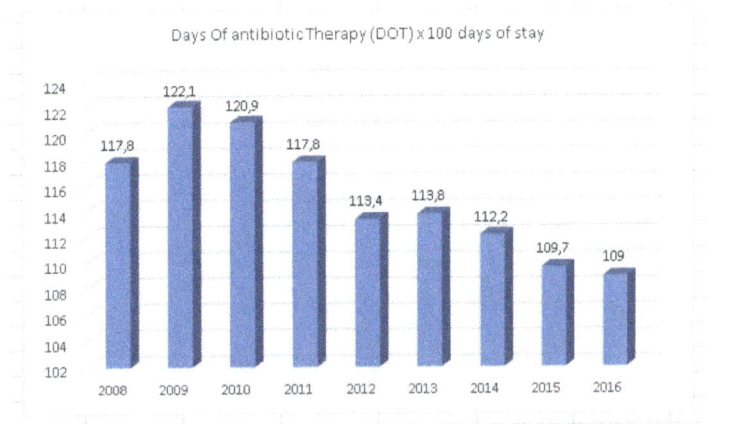

Figure 7. Reduction in the use of days of antibiotic treatment (DOT) for 100 stays in the recent years.

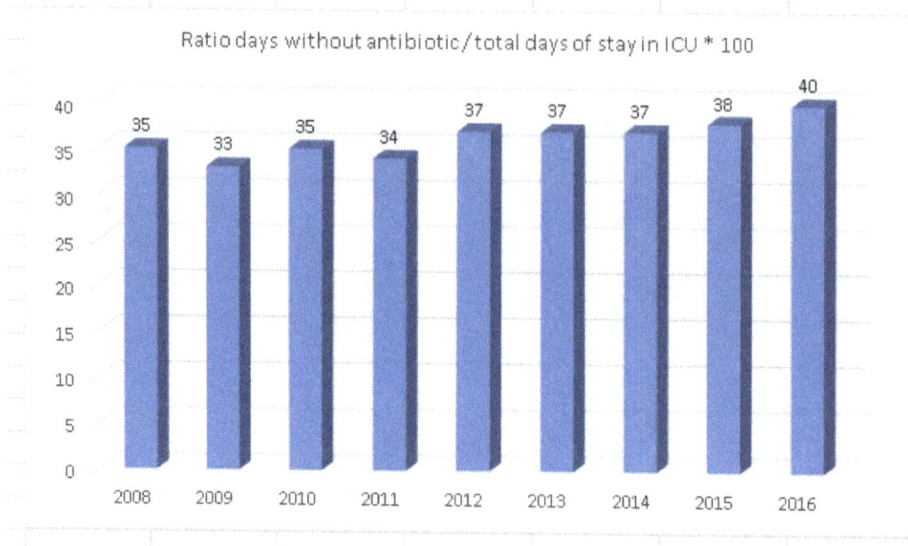

Figure 8. Increase in the number of days in the ICU without antibiotic treatment over the years.

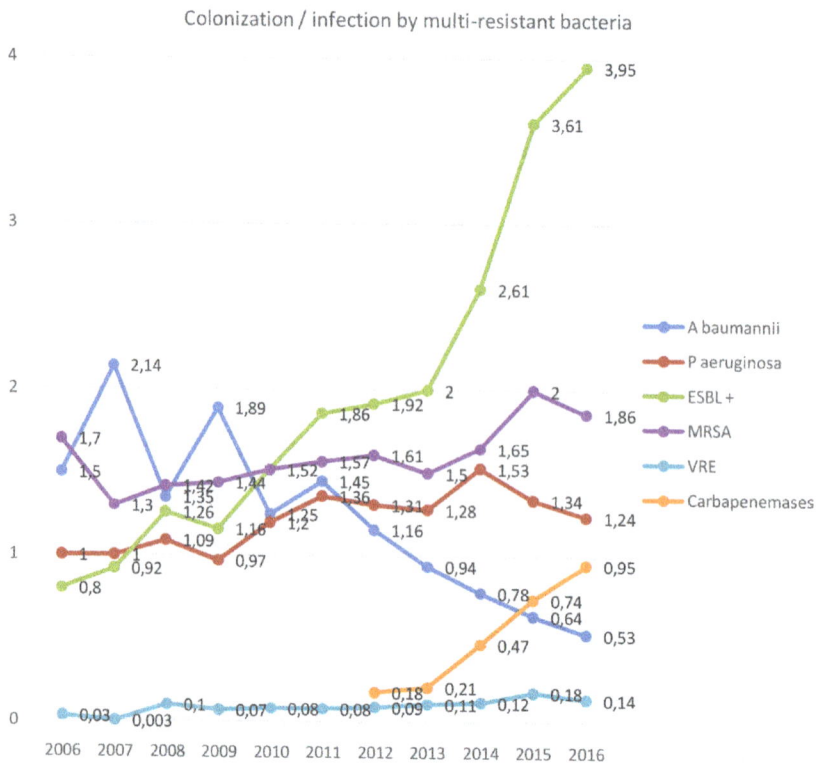

Figure 9. Infection/colonization by MRB. ENVIN study in the interval 2006–2016.

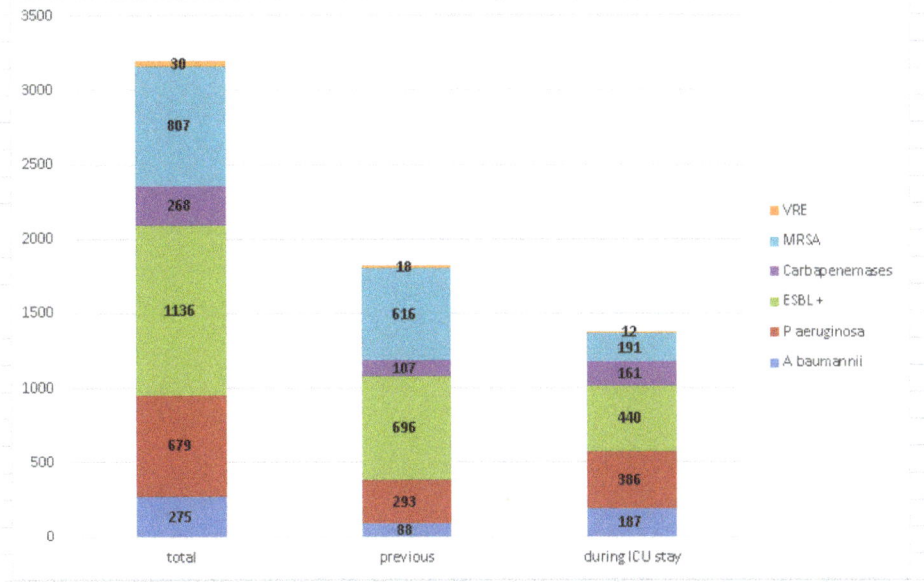

Figure 10. Isolation of MR germs in the RZ period globally, upon admission and during their stay in the ICU.

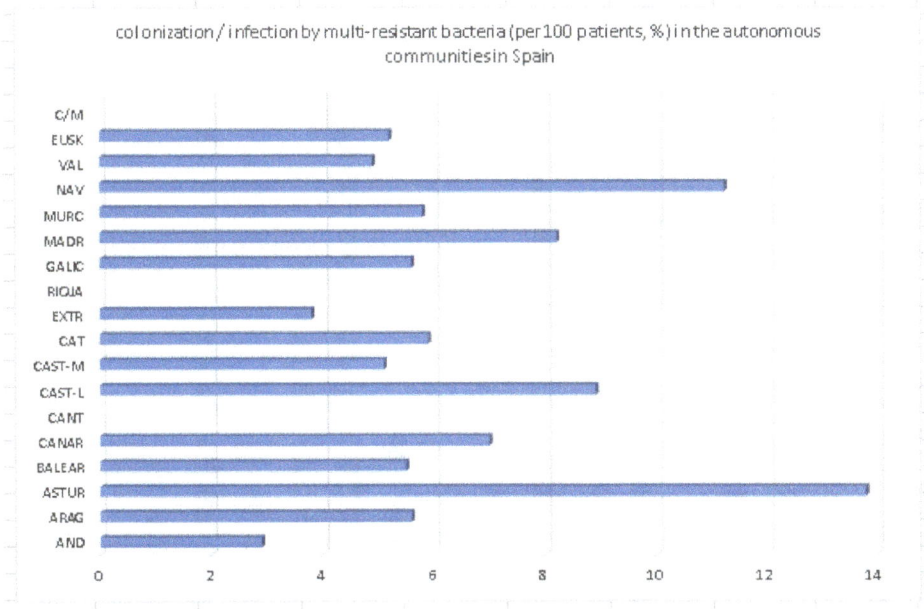

Figure 11. Isolation rate in the different autonomous communities. AND Andalucia, ARAG Aragón, ASTUR Asturias, BALEAR Balearic Islands, CANAR Canary Islands, CAST-L Castilla-León, CAST-M Castilla-La Mancha, CAT Catalonia, EXTR Extremadura, RIOJA La RIOJA, GALIC Galicia, MADR Madrid, MURC Murcia, NAV Navarra, VAL Valencian community, EUSK Euskadi, C/M Ceuta/Melilla.

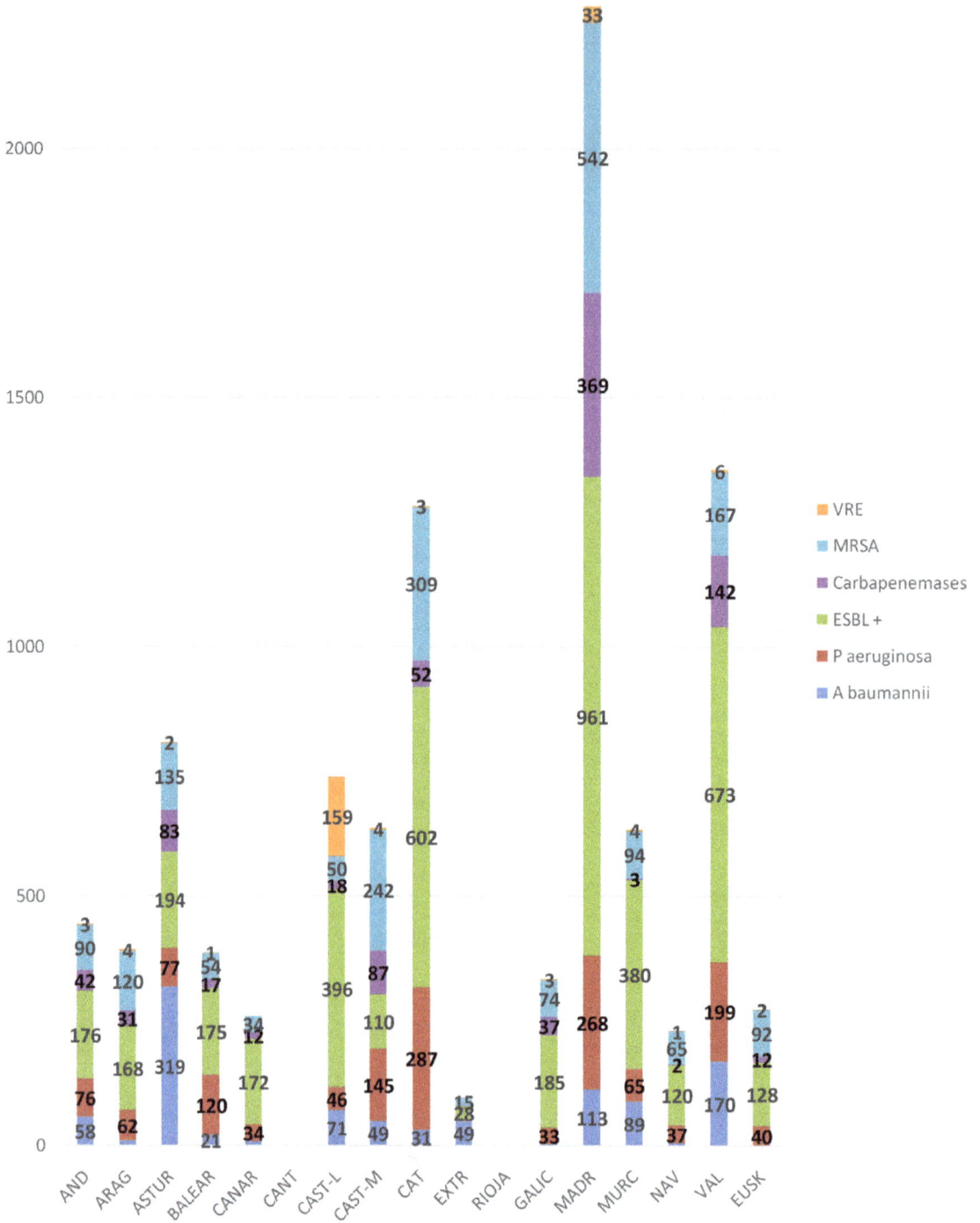

Figure 12. Heterogeneity of MRB isolates, counting colonizations and infections, during the period of RZ study. In most autonomous communities, the most frequent type of MRB is ESBL producing GNB. The presence of *A. baumannii* has become much less frequent, except in Extremadura and Asturias. In the Canary Islands, there are 0 VRE isolates; in Extremadura, there are zero isolates of VRE, one isolation of carbapenemase producing germ and three isolates of *P. aeruginosa*; there are few isolates of *A. baumannii* in Aragón [9], Canary Islands [8], Galicia [3] and Navarra [5]; and finally there is no isolation (0) of *A. baumannii* in Euskadi.

5. Data of the ICU of the hospital of Sagunto

Our unit starts the data collection in the ENVIN project the same year of its beginning (1994). We started the RZ project in April 2014, and until now (January 2018) have followed the guidelines of the RZ project in the prevention and management of patients with MRB. We reported 195 isolates in 179 patients for 46 months, with 1966 admissions and a rate of 9.1 patients with MRB/100 admissions (**Figure 13**).

In our unit, a high prevalence of *A. baumannii* was initially observed, without a clear seasonal profile. Over time, there is a decrease in *A. baumannii* and an increase in the ESBL carrier

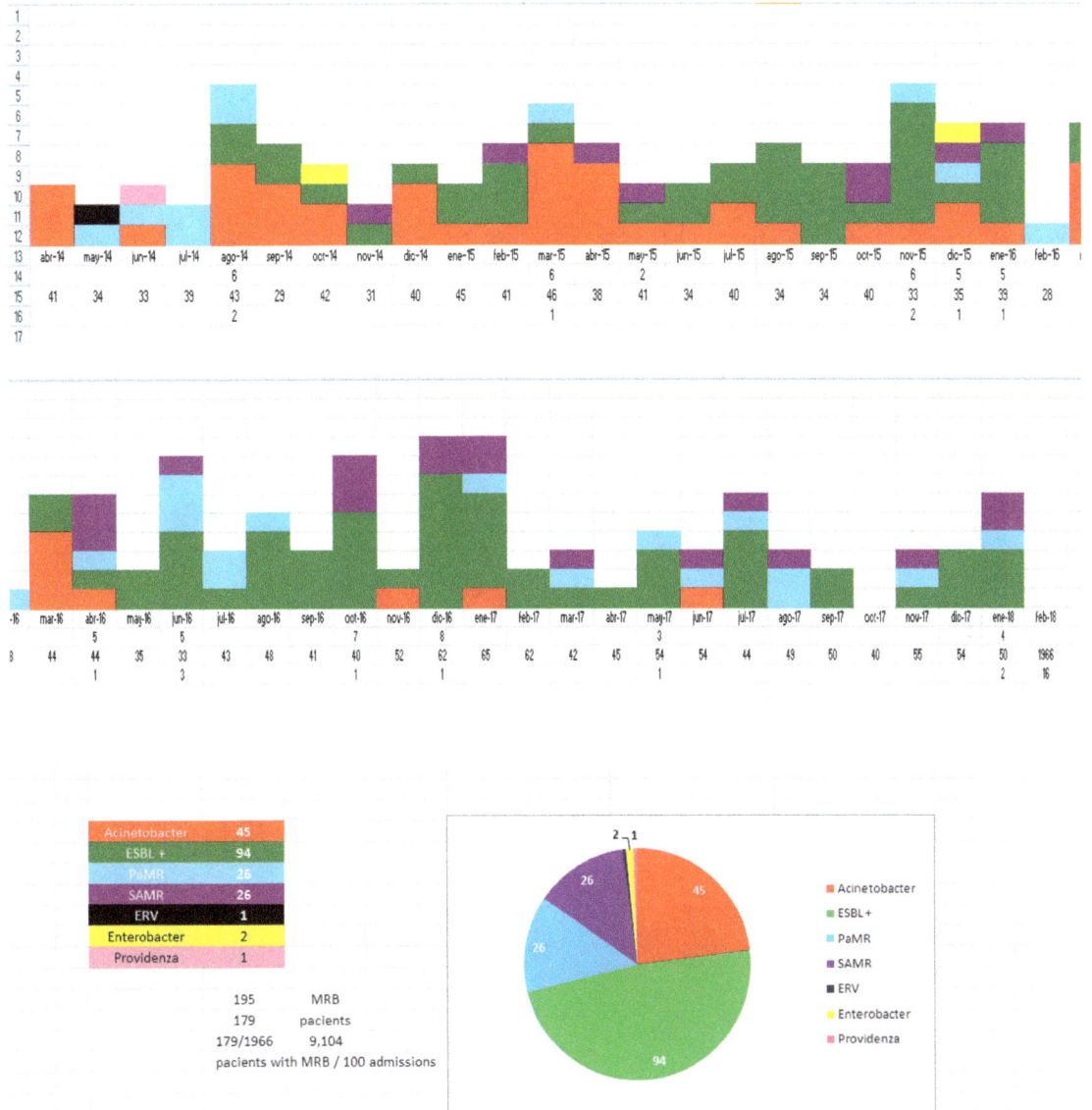

Figure 13. Occurrence of MRB in our ICU Fromm the beginning of RZ project until February 2018. Acinetobacter supposes globally a 25% of isolates, with a rate of 50% of ESBL producer germs.

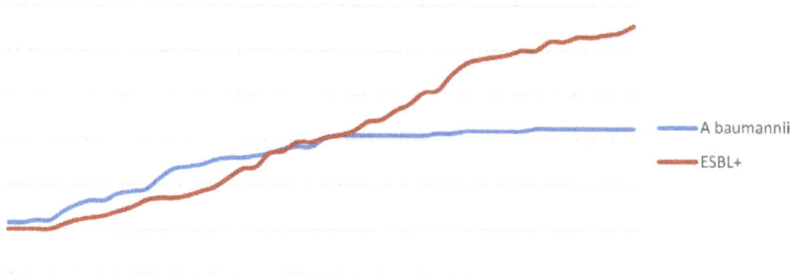

Figure 14. Accumulated frequency of colonized and infected patients by *A. baumannii* and ESBL producer germs.

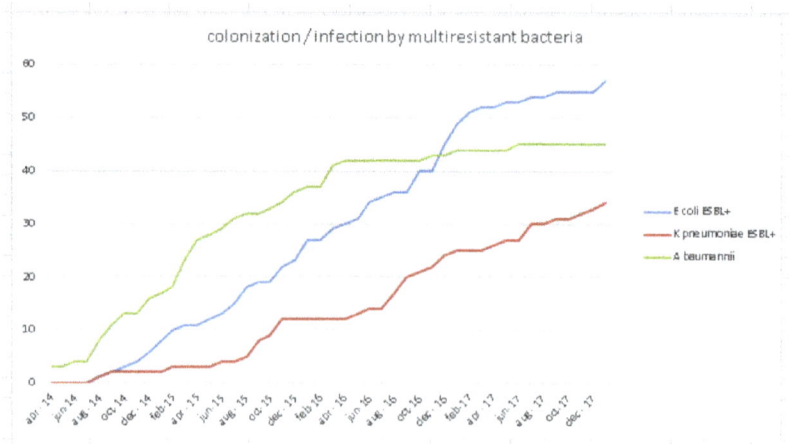

Figure 15. Accumulated frequency of colonized and infected patients by the most frequently isolated germs in the ICU of the hospital of Sagunto.

Figure 16. Indicators of the RZ project at the local (hospital of Sagunto), regional (Valencian community) and national (Spain) levels.

Relación de Bacterias Multirresistentes al ingreso y durante el ingreso

UNIDAD	N	%	COMUNIDAD VALENCIANA	N	%	NACIONAL	N	%
SARM (MRSA)	12	10,08	SARM (MRSA)	433	21,46	SARM (MRSA)	3230	21,20
Enterococo resistente Vancomicina	1	0,84	Enterococo resistente Vancomicina	9	0,45	Enterococo resistente Vancomicina	273	1,79
Pseudomonas multirresistente	13	10,92	Pseudomonas multirresistente	337	16,70	Pseudomonas multirresistente	2560	16,80
Acinetobacter R-Imipenem	42	35,29	Acinetobacter R-Imipenem	212	10,51	Acinetobacter R-Imipenem	1397	9,17
Enterobacteria - BLEE	51	42,86	Enterobacteria - BLEE	859	42,57	Enterobacteria - BLEE	6396	41,98
BGN - Carbapenemasa	0	0,00	BGN - Carbapenemasa	168	8,33	BGN - Carbapenemasa	1380	9,06
TOTAL	119		TOTAL	2018		TOTAL	15236	

Relación de Bacterias Multirresistentes durante el ingreso incluyendo colonización e infección

UNIDAD	N	%	COMUNIDAD VALENCIANA	N	%	NACIONAL	N	%
SARM (MRSA)	0	0,00	SARM (MRSA)	113	11,36	SARM (MRSA)	731	11,46
Enterococo resistente Vancomicina	0	0,00	Enterococo resistente Vancomicina	3	0,30	Enterococo resistente Vancomicina	114	1,79
Pseudomonas multirresistente	3	10,00	Pseudomonas multirresistente	217	21,81	Pseudomonas multirresistente	1472	23,08
Acinetobacter R-Imipenem	19	63,33	Acinetobacter R-Imipenem	139	13,97	Acinetobacter R-Imipenem	948	14,86
Enterobacteria - BLEE	8	26,67	Enterobacteria - BLEE	403	40,50	Enterobacteria - BLEE	2365	37,08
BGN - Carbapenemasa	0	0,00	BGN - Carbapenemasa	120	12,06	BGN - Carbapenemasa	748	11,73
TOTAL	30		TOTAL	995		TOTAL	6378	

Relación de Bacterias Multirresistentes durante el ingreso solo infección

UNIDAD	N	%	COMUNIDAD VALENCIANA	N	%	NACIONAL	N	%
SARM (MRSA)	0	0,00	SARM (MRSA)	18	6,19	SARM (MRSA)	316	11,72
Enterococo resistente Vancomicina	0	0,00	Enterococo resistente Vancomicina	2	0,69	Enterococo resistente Vancomicina	23	0,85
Pseudomonas multirresistente	1	33,33	Pseudomonas multirresistente	102	35,05	Pseudomonas multirresistente	830	30,79
Acinetobacter R-Imipenem	2	66,67	Acinetobacter R-Imipenem	46	15,81	Acinetobacter R-Imipenem	403	14,95
Enterobacteria - BLEE	0	0,00	Enterobacteria - BLEE	99	34,02	Enterobacteria - BLEE	881	32,68
BGN - Carbapenemasa	0	0,00	BGN - Carbapenemasa	24	8,25	BGN - Carbapenemasa	243	9,01
TOTAL	3		TOTAL	291		TOTAL	2696	

Figure 17. MRB isolated at admission and during their stay, such as colonization or infection, at the local, regional and national levels.

bacteria, and a slowly increasing incidence of MRSA and *P. aeruginosa* (**Figure 13**). Assessing the cumulative incidence, there is a catch-up of the ESBL + germs to the initially predominant Acinetobacter at the end of 2015–beginning of 2016 (**Figure 14**); if we separate the ESBL + germs, the highest cumulative frequency of E coli than of *A. baumannii* is observed at the end of 2016. In the last months also, the frequency of occurrence of *K. pneumoniae* is higher than that of *A. baumannii* (**Figure 15**).

During the RZ project, in our unit, 80 MRB were detected on admission and 26 during stay; this implies a global estimate, during the entire project period, of 6.29 patients with BMR at admission for every 100 admitted patients, and 2.04 patients with BMR during their stay in ICU per 100 patients admitted and 5.72 patients for 1000 stays. The income indicator is significantly higher than that of the Valencian Community (2.22%) and the national one (2.62%); and the indicators during their income are only slightly larger than the regional (1.87 and 4.28‰) and national (1.82 and 3.36‰) estimates (**Figure 16**). There have only been three nosocomial infections for BMR acquired in ICU during this RZ period, 1 for Pa and 2 for Ab, with a BMR infection rate acquired in ICU lower (0.24 per 100 patients admitted to ICU) than the regional (0.60%) and the national rates (0.79%).

The profile of germs is different: predominance in our unit of germs producing ESBL + (42.8%) and *A. baumannii* (35.3%), with a lower presence of *P. aeruginosa* (10.9%) and MRSA (10.1%). %); while at the regional and national level, the most common germs in decreasing order are Enterobacteria ESBL + (42.6% regional and 42% national), MRSA (21.5 and 21.2%), *P. aeruginosa* (16.7 and 16.8%), *A. baumannii* (10.5 and 9.2%) and GNB producers of carbapenemases (8.3 and 9.1%) (**Figure 17**).

6. Conclusions

The problem of multidrug resistance is serious. The loss of efficacy of antibiotics, within our current technified medicine, would limit procedures such as transplants, complex surgeries, the management of cancer patients, and so on. It is the responsibility of EVERYBODY to make an efficient use of antibiotics. We must remember that a large part of the use of these molecules is done at the industrial level, out of sanitary management.

The striking finding of the NORTH-SOUTH and WEST-EAST gradient of MRB isolates frequency can have several explanations: different policies of antibiotic use, environmental conditions (heat) that favors the persistence of certain germs in the hospital environment, variable culture of security within the hospital centers, and so on.

The RZ project, despite the difficulties in its development, shows efficacy in reducing MRB infections acquired in the ICU. It has been achieved up to 40% of the days in ICU without the use of antibiotics. The number of germs discovered at the time of admission is greater than during the stay in ICU. The MRBs that caused colonization acquired in ICU increased, while the infections acquired by BMR decreased. A great proportion of MRSA and ESBL among isolated microorganisms has been documented on admission, and germs producers of carbapenemases, *P. aeruginosa* and *A. baumannii* are more frequent during their stay in the ICU. There are important differences between autonomous communities; there may even be differences between different units of critics of the same hospital. The active search for MRB in patients at the time of admission has doubled its detection. The application of the recommended measures in RZ has achieved to reduce acquired MRB infections acquired up to 45%.

Author details

Miguel Ángel García García[1]*, Alfonso Martínez Cornejo[1], David Arizo León[1] and María Ángeles Rosero Arenas[2]

*Address all correspondence to: mangelesymangel@gmail.com

1 Intensive Care Unit, Hospital de Sagunto, Valencia, Spain

2 Primary Care, Cheste, Valencia, Spain

References

[1] US Department of Health and Human Services. Centers for Disease Control and Prevention. Antibiotic Resistance Threats in the United States. 20th February, 2018. Available from: https://www.cdc.gov/drugresistance/threat-report-2013/index.html

[2] European Centre for Disease Prevention and Control. Healthcare–associated infections acquired in intensive care units. In: ECDC Annual Epidemiological Report for 2015.

Stockholm: ECDC; 2017. Available from: https://ecdc.europa.eu/sites/portal/files/documents/AER_for_2015-healthcare-associated-infections.pdf

[3] Fridkin SK, Welbel SF, Weinstein RA. Magnitude and prevention of nosocomial infections in the intensive care unit. Infectious Disease Clinics of North America. 1997;**11**:479

[4] Vincent JL, Rello J, Marshall J, et al. International study of the prevalence and outcomes of infection in intensive care units. Journal of the American Medical Association. 2009; **302**:2323

[5] Hynes-Gay P, Lalla P, Leo M, et al. Understanding sepsis: From SIRS to septic shock. Dynamics (Pembroke, Ontario). 2002;**13**:17

[6] Rice LB. Federal funding for the study of antimicrobial resistance in nosocomial pathogens: No ESKAPE. The Journal of Infectious Diseases. 2008;**197**:1079

[7] McDonald LC, Banerjee SN, Jarvis WR. Seasonal variation of acinetobacter infections: 1987-1996. Nosocomial Infections Surveillance System. Clinical Infectious Diseases. 1999;**29**:1133

[8] Sheppard FR, Keiser P, Craft DW, et al. The majority of US combat casualty soft-tissue wounds are not infected or colonized upon arrival or during treatment at a continental US military medical facility. American Journal of Surgery. 2010;**200**:489

[9] Siempos II, Vardakas KZ, Kyriakopoulos CE, et al. Predictors of mortality in adult patients with ventilator-associated pneumonia: A meta-analysis. Shock. 2010;**33**:590

[10] Davis JS, McMillan M, Swaminathan A, et al. A 16-year prospective study of community-onset bacteriemic Acinetobacter pneumonia: Low mortality with appropriate initial empirical antibiotic protocols. Chest. 2014;**146**:1038

[11] Marchaim D, Chopra T, Bhargava A, et al. Recent exposure to antimicrobials and carbapenem-resistant Enterobacteriaceae: The role of antimicrobial stewardship. Infection Control and Hospital Epidemiology. 2012;**33**:817

[12] Neidell MJ, Cohen B, Furuya Y, et al. Costs of healthcare- and community-associated infections with antimicrobial-resistant versus antimicrobial-susceptible organisms. Clinical Infectious Diseases. 2012;**55**:807

[13] Paul M, Shani V, Muchtar E, et al. Systematic review and meta-analysis of the efficacy of appropriate empiric therapy for sepsis. Antimicrobial Agents and Chemotherapy. 2010;**55**:807

[14] Kollef MH, Fraser VJ. Antibiotic resistance in the intensive care unit. Annals of Internal Medicine. 2001;**134**:298

[15] Climo MW, Yokoe DS, Warren DK, et al. Effect of daily chlorhexidine bathing on hospital-adquired infection. The New England Journal of Medicine. 2013;**368**:533

[16] Goossens H, Ferech M, Vander Stichele R, et al. Outpatient antibiotic use in Europe and association with resistance: A cross-national database study. Lancet. 2005;**365**:579-587

[17] Pechère JC. Rotating antibiotics in the intensive care unit: Feasible, apparently beneficial, but questions remain. Critical Care. 2002;**6**:9

[18] European Centre for Disease Prevention and Control. Surveillance of antimicrobial resistance in Europe 2016. In: Annual Report of the European Antimicrobial Resistance Network (EARS-Net). Stockholm: ECDC; 2017

Aneurysmal Subarachnoid Hemorrhage

Adel E. Ahmed Ganaw, Abdulgafoor M. Tharayil,
Ali O. Mohamed Bel Khair, Saher Tahseen,
Jazib Hassan,
Mohammad Faisal Abdullah Malmstrom and
Sohel Mohamed Gamal Ahmed

Abstract

Aneurysmal subarachnoid hemorrhage (SAH) is a devastating neurological syndrome, which occurs at a rate of 3–25 per 100,000 population. Smoking and hypertension are the most important risk factors of subarachnoid hemorrhage. Rupture of cerebral aneurysm leads to rapid spread of blood into cerebrospinal fluid and subsequently leads to sudden increase of intracranial pressure and severe headache. Subarachnoid hemorrhage is associated with neurological (such as re-bleeding and vasospasm) and systemic (such as myocardial injury and hyponatremia) complications that are causes of high mortality and morbidity. Although patients with poor-grade subarachnoid hemorrhage are at higher risk of neurological and systemic complications, the early and aggressive management of this group of patient has decreased overall mortality by 17% in last 40 years. Early aneurysm repair, close monitoring in dedicated neurological intensive care unit, prevention, and aggressive management of medical and neurological complications are the most important strategies to improve outcome.

Keywords: albumin, aneurysmal subarachnoid hemorrhage, vasospasm, re-bleeding, hyponatremia, cardiac complication, coiling, clipping

1. Introduction

Subarachnoid hemorrhage (SAH) is a devastating disease and is associated with high mortality and poor outcomes among survivors, management by multidisciplinary team is associated with improved outcomes; however, intensive care management presents big challenge. Most of spontaneous SAH is due to the rupture of saccular aneurysm, the prevalence of intracranial saccular aneurysm by radiographic and autopsy series is 5%, about 20–30% of patients have several aneurysms [1].

Aneurysmal SAH (aSAH) occurs at a rate of 2–16 per 100,000 population, mostly occurring between 40 and 60 years of age; however, young children and elderly can be affected. The incidence of SAH is higher in women than men, which may be due to hormonal status. African Americans are at a higher risk of SAH than Caucasian Americans. Mortality rate is about 60% within first 6 months [2, 3].

2. Circle of Willis

The circle of Willis is an anastomotic structure. It is formed when the internal carotid artery enters the cranial cavity bilaterally and divides into the anterior cerebral artery and middle cerebral artery, and the anterior cerebral arteries are then united by an anterior communicating artery. These anastomoses form the anterior half of the circle (anterior circulation). Posteriorly, the basilar artery branches to give left and right posterior cerebral artery (posterior circulation). Posterior cerebral arteries join the internal carotid system anteriorly to complete the circle via posterior communicating arteries. **Figure 1** shows the common sites of cerebral aneurysm [4, 5].

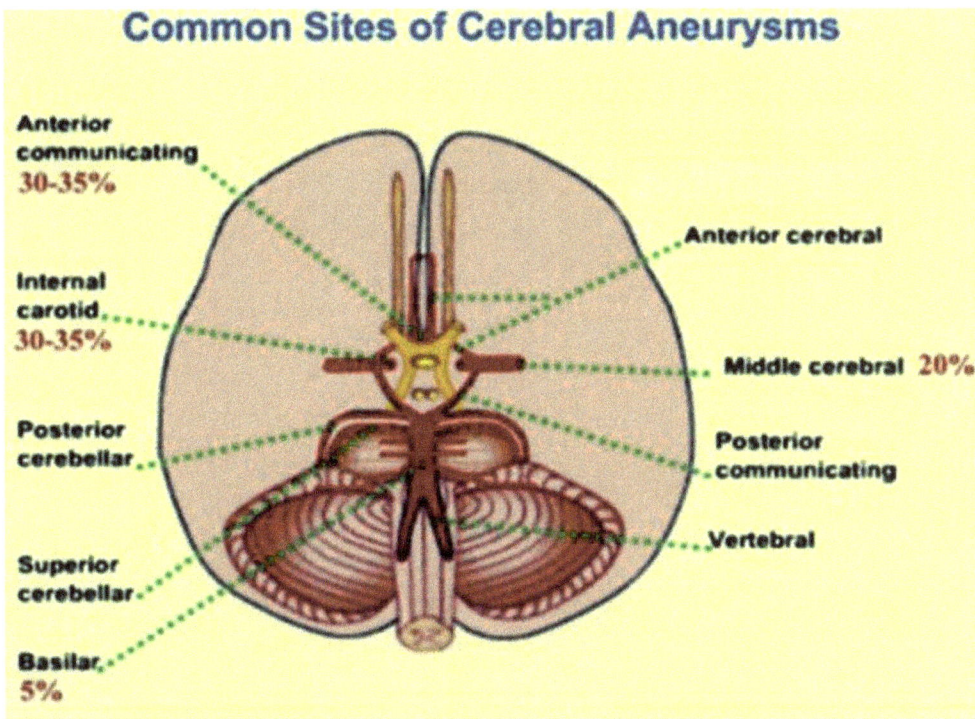

Figure 1. Common sites of cerebral aneurysm [5].

3. Etiology

Subarachnoid hemorrhage is defined as bleeding into the space between the arachnoid and pia mater of the meninges enclosing the brain (subarachnoid space). The most common reason for spontaneous (non-traumatic) SAH is the rupture of a cerebral aneurysm (85%) [5].

In about 15% of non-traumatic SAH, no bleeding cause is identified by digital subtraction angiography (DSA). In these scenarios, differentiation between perimesencephalic and non-perimesencephalic location of the SAH is very important to determine further therapeutic approach [3].

Perimesencephalic SAH (PMSAH) is defined by the absence of an aneurysmatic bleeding and the classic presence of blood within the perimesencephalic and prepontine cisterns [3].

Computed topography angiogram (CTA) and magnetic resonance angiography (MRA) have high sensitivity of excluding aneurysmal bleedings in PMSAH.

PMSAH has less complication and better prognosis than aneurysmal SAH.

Non-perimesencephalic is SAH without bleeding source in the baseline DSA, the chance of positive findings in a follow-up angiography fluctuated between 5 and 35%, that is why DSA should be repeated not before 3 weeks after the initial bleeding if there are no other therapeutic indications [3].

Non-traumatic SAH can be caused by various other non-aneurysmatic causes (**Table 1**), and the management of these cases must be performed according to the underlying cause [3].

Disease	Example
Infectious arterial vasculitis	Mycotic (infectious) aneurysm
	Meningovascular lues
	Lyme disease
	Gnathostomiasis (Gnathostoma spinigerum)
Immune vasculitis	Primary CNS angiitis
	Polyarteritis nodosa
	Wegener's vasculitis
	Churg-Strauss syndrome
	Behçet's disease
Other cerebrovascular diseases	Arteriovenous angioma
	Dural arteriovenous fistula
	Spinal arterial aneurysm
	Intracranial arterial dissection
	Venous sinus thrombosis
	Cerebral amyloid angiopathy
	Moyamoya disease

Disease	Example
Tumor	Intracranial und intraspinal tumor
Hematology	Sickle cell anemia
Drugs	Anticoagulants and thrombolytic therapy
Substance abuse	Cocaine

Table 1. Rare causes of non-traumatic SAH [3].

4. Risk factors

Most spontaneous SAHs result from the rupture of intracranial aneurysms; therefore, risk factors for aneurysm formation overlap with risk factors for SAH.

(1) Cigarette smoking: It is associated with 11-fold increased risk of SAH. Worldwide, it is the most important preventable risk factor, which has been proved in numerous cohort (relative risk, RR, of current smoking, 2.2) and case-control studies (odds ratio, OR, 3.1); cigarette smoking also hastened aneurysm growth rate [2, 3].

(2) Hypertension: It is a major risk factor for SAH and possibly for aneurysm formation and fatal aneurysm rupture. Treatment of hypertension may reduce the risk of aneurysmal SAH [6].

(3) Alcohol abuse: Excessive alcohol abuse raises the possibility for SAH independent of cigarette smoking, age, and history of hypertension [3].

(4) Genetic risk: The risk of SAH increases seven folds in first-degree relatives of patient; in addition, number of rare inherited conditions (Autosomal dominant polycystic kidney, Ehler-Danlos syndrome) are associated with cerebral aneurysm and SAH [2, 6].

(5) Use of sympathomimetic drugs such as (cocaine) [6].

(6) Female sex: This is believed to be due to estrogen deficiency (estrogen replacement therapy reduces the risk), so it is higher in postmenopausal women than premenopausal ones [3, 6].

(7) Antithrombotic therapy: It increases the severity of the hemorrhage, there are no data to prove whether antithrombotic therapy increases the risk of aneurysmal rupture or not [3, 6].

(8) Inflammation seems to play a vital role in the pathogenesis and growth of intracranial aneurysms. Prominent mediators include the nuclear factor k - light-chain enhancer of activated B cells (NF-κB), tumor necrosis factor, macrophages, and reactive oxygen species. Although there are no controlled studies in humans, 3-hydroxy-3-methylglutaryl coenzyme A reductase inhibitors (statins) and calcium channel blockers could impede aneurysm formation by the inhibition of NF-κB and other pathways [6, 7].

(9) Aneurysm size of 7 mm increases risk of rupture and subsequent SAH [6].

(10) Aneurysm morphology such as bottleneck shape and the ratio of size of aneurysm to par-ent vessels are associated with rupture of aneurysm [6].

(11) The risk of SAH increases in symptomatic patient with large unruptured cerebral aneu-rysm especially if it is located either on posterior communicating artery or on the verte-brobasilar system [6].

5. Pathophysiology

Smoking, chronic hypertension, and alcohol abuse lead to weakened arterial tunica media. Chronic exposure to intravascular shear stress leads to pouching of the weakened wall, espe-cially in the vicinity of bifurcations where turbulent flow is prominent.

The aneurysmal rupture is directly proportional to the size of the aneurysm, which is rising from 0.05% in aneurysms less than 10 mm to 6% for those greater than 25 mm.

More than 80% of cerebral aneurysm arises from the anterior carotid circulation (anterior and posterior communicating and middle cerebral arteries), with only 10–20% arising from the posterior vertebrobasilar circulation [1, 2].

Subsequent to aneurysmal rupture, blood spreads quickly within cerebrospinal fluid (CSF), rapidly increasing intracranial pressure (ICP), this sudden increase in the ICP leads to severe headache, cerebral edema, and hydrocephalus. Bleeding usually lasts for a few seconds; however, re-bleeding is common and occurs within the first 24 h. The presence of blood and breakdown products of hemoglobin in the subarachnoid space is responsible for meningeal irritation, meningism, and vasospasm [2].

6. Clinical manifestation

Headache is the hallmark of aSAH in awake patient who describes it "as worst headache in their life," this headache has a sudden onset and immediately reaches maximal inten-sity (thunderclap headache). Sentinel headache is also reported by 10–43% of patients, which is minor headache, and it is symptoms of minor hemorrhage (sentinel bleed or warning leak). Most of these minor hemorrhages occur within 2–8 weeks before major hemorrhage [6, 8].

The headache may be associated with nausea and/or vomiting, stiff neck, photophobia, brief loss of consciousness, or focal neurological deficits (including cranial nerve palsies).

Seizures occur in about 26% of patients within the first 24 h of SAH, most of the time before medical care is accessed. It is common in presence of intracerebral hemorrhage, in hypertensive patients, and patient with middle cerebral or anterior communicating artery aneurysms [6].

7. Diagnosis

7.1. Non-contrast head CT scan

Non-contrast CT scan is the cornerstone of SAH diagnosis, it confirms the presence of blood clot in subarachnoid space in most of the cases if the scan is performed in the first 24 h, and it may also provide an idea of the cause of the bleeding and site of the aneurysm. In addition to that, it is useful in diagnosis of intraventricular and subdural hematoma [2, 6].

CT scan sensitivity is highest in the first 3 days (close to 100%) and progressively decreases over time to about 58% in the fifth day [6].

7.2. Lumbar puncture

The typical findings are an elevated opening pressure and presence of xanthochromia, which can last for 2 weeks after SAH. Xanthochromia represents hemoglobin degradation products in CSF and indicates that the blood has been in CSF for at least 2 h [6, 9].

7.3. Brain MRI

MRI has advantages over CT brain in detection of subacute subarachnoid hemorrhage (after 4 days), when head CT scan is negative and there is clinical suspicion of SAH, and possibly avoiding the need of lumbar puncture. The most important disadvantages are difficulty in scanning acutely confused ill patient, without sedation for at least 45 minutes, predisposing to motion artifact, and is expensive in comparison with CT [6].

7.4. Digital subtraction angiography (DSA)

Once diagnosis of SAH has been completed, the source of bleeding must be identified with angiographic studies. Digital subtraction angiography (DSA) is the gold standard for the detection of intracranial aneurysm and study of anatomical features of cerebral blood vessels [3, 6].

7.5. CT and MR angiography

Both CT and MR angiography are useful for screening and pre-surgical planning, they can detect aneurysms ≥3 mm with high degree of sensitivity; however, they are less sensitive than conventional angiography. CTA can be achieved immediately after the diagnosis of SAH by CT scan when the patient is still in scanner; CTA is more practical than MRA in acute setting. CTA is used as an alternative to conventional angiography in SAH patients, especially in acute setting and rapidly declining patient who needs emergent craniotomy for hematoma evacuation. CTA can substitute catheter cerebral angiography in older patient with degenerative vascular disease provided that the quality is excellent and investigation is performed cautiously. Negative CTA should be followed by two- and three-dimensional cerebral angiography in case of diffuse SAH [3, 6]. MRA is rarely indicated in SAH, because of limited routine availability, difficulty in scanning acutely sick patient, who is poorly compliant to commands, which can affect quality of the study, moreover MRA is time consuming and very expensive [6].

8. Grading of SAH

Hard work has been made for the development of scales to clinically grade patients with SAH, to assess the severity of initial injury, to guide treatment decision, to provide prognostic information regarding outcome, and to standardize patient evaluation for scientific study purposes. Since 1933, more than 40 grading systems have been proposed for patients with cerebral aneurysm. Currently, the most commonly used SAH grading scales are the Hunt and Hess scale, Fisher scale, Glasgow Coma Scale (GCS), and the World Federation of Neurological Surgeons (WFNS) scale [10].

8.1. World Federation of Neurosurgeons SAH Scale (WFNS)

In 1998, an expert judgment committee projected the WFNS scale, it was based on GCS and the presence of focal neurological deficit (**Table 2**). Numerous studies found direct association between WFNS grade and outcome [10].

WFNS scale	GCS	Motor deficit, aphasia±hemiparesis or hemiplegia
I	15	Absent
II	14–13	Absent
III	14–13	Present
IV	12–7	Present/absent
V	6–3	Present/absent

Table 2. World Federation of Neurosurgeons SAH scale.

8.2. Prognosis on Admission of Aneurysmal Subarachnoid Hemorrhage (PAASH)

PAASH is solely based on the GCS; it has excellent internal and external validity in regard to clinical outcome. In a study comparing prognostic accuracy of WFNS and PAASH, PAASH had a good prognostic value for patient outcome (**Table 3**) [3].

Scale	Grade	Criteria	Proportion of patient with poor outcome (%)
WFNS	I	GCS 15	14.8
	II	GCS 13–14 no focal deficits	29.4
	III	GCS 13–14 focal deficits	52.6
	IV	GCS 7–12	58.3
	V	GCS 3–6	92.7
PAASH	I	GCS 15	14.8
	II	GCS 11–14	41.3
	III	GCS 8–10	74.4
	IV	GCS 4–7	84.7
	V	GCS 3	93.9

Table 3. Two SAH grading scales with criteria per grade and relation with outcome [3].

8.3. The Hunt and Hess scale

The Hunt and Hess scale was projected in 1968 as an adjustment to an older system initially described by Botterell and colleagues in 1956. The scale was prepared to stratify the surgical risk and to help the surgeon on making appropriate decision in appropriate time. It is well known in the neuroscientific community; however, many of the terms used to define grades, such as drowsy, stupor or deep coma, headache (mild, moderate, severe), nuchal rigidity (slight vs. sever), are subjective and vague which makes this grading system neither reliable nor valid (**Table 4**) [3, 10].

Grade	Clinical description
I	Asymptomatic or minimal headache and slight nuchal rigidity.
II	Moderate to severe headache, nuchal rigidity, no neurological deficit other than cranial nerve palsy.
III	Drowsiness, confusion, or mild focal deficit.
IV	Stupor, moderate to severe hemiparesis, and possibly decerebrate rigidity and vegetative disturbances.
V	Deep coma, decerebrate rigidity, moribund appearance.

Table 4. Hunt and Hess scale.

8.4. Fisher scale

In 1980, the Fisher scale was projected to predict cerebral vasospasm after SAH (**Figure 2**), the scale quantifies the amount of blood seen on CT scan (**Table 5**). It was developed when imaging technology had roughly one-tenth of the resolution currently available. Subarachnoid

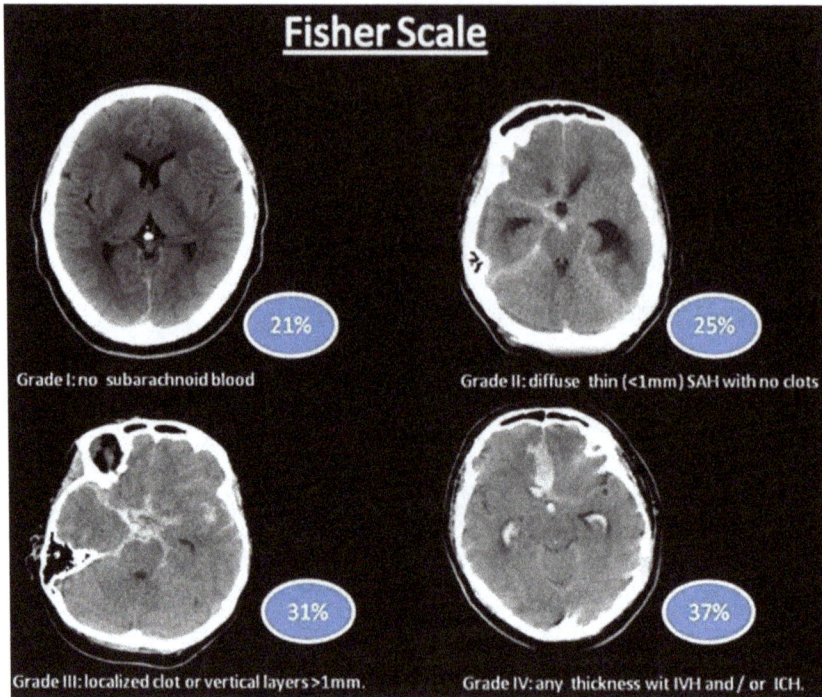

Figure 2. Scale grading system used to quantify the amount of subarachnoid hemorrhage and intraventricular hemorrhage (IVH). The percentages in the circles refer to the risk of vasospasm. Grades III and IV in the scale are the ones with the higher risk to develop "symptomatic vasospasm." Adopted with permission from Ref. [11].

Group	Blood on CT scan
I	No subarachnoid detected.
II	Diffuse or thin vertical layer <1 mm thick.
III	Localized subarachnoid clot and/or vertical layer >1 mm thick.
IV	Intraventricular or intra-parenchymal clot with diffuse or no SAH.

Table 5. Fisher grade scale.

clot less than 1 mm in true thickness is uncommon, as is the finding of no blood on admission CT scan, therefore, grades 1 and 2 were actually be quite uncommon [3, 10].

9. Complications associated with SAH

Complications of subarachnoid hemorrhage can be divided into CNS and systemic complications.

9.1. CNS complications

Re-bleeding, vasospasm, hydrocephalus, and seizures are the most important CNS complications of SAH. The high rates of mortality and morbidity after aneurysmal subarachnoid hemorrhage are mainly due to CNS complications.

9.1.1. Re-bleeding

Re-bleeding occurs at a rate of 4–13% in the first 24 h, maximal risk of re-bleeding is in the first 2–12 h, most of re-bleeding (73%) occurs within the first 72 h of initial hemorrhage. Re-bleeding is associated with very high mortality and morbidity, especially if it occurs in the first 12 h after the hemorrhage, the mortality rate reaches to 70% [6, 12].

Many factors are considered as predictor for re-bleeding:

Hunt-Hess grade on admission.

Maximal aneurysmal diameter.

High initial blood pressure.

Sentinel headache preceding SAH.

Longer interval from ictus to admission.

Ventriculostomy before aneurysmal treatment [6, 13].

Re-bleeding diagnosis is based on the deterioration of neurological status and appearance of new hemorrhage in CT scan. Early securing of the aneurysm is the treatment of choice to prevent re-bleeding; however, the optimum time for early intervention is unclear whether intervention within 24 h (ultra-early) is superior to intervention after 3 days [12].

The management of high blood pressure after SAH is still debatable due to the lack of evidence from randomized controlled trial. Data from observational studies propose that aggressive management of blood pressure reduces the risk of re-bleeding, however, at the expense of an increase in secondary ischemia. It looks acceptable but without strong evidence to stop all antihypertensive medications that the patients were taking, and treat hypertension only when it is extremely high. It is very difficult to give limits for extreme blood pressures, because extreme varies between patients and it is affected by many factors such as previous blood pressure, cardiac disease, patient age, and other factors [3].

European stroke organization guidelines for the management of intracranial aneurysm and subarachnoid hemorrhage recommended that the systolic blood pressure should be kept less than 180 mmHg in patients with unsecured aneurysm, till the aneurysm is secured with coiling or clipping. They also recommended keeping mean arterial pressure (MAP) above 90 mmHg when blood pressure is lowered [3].

Nicardipine is short-acting calcium channel blocker, used for smooth control of blood pressure [3, 6].

For patient with an unavoidable delay in obliteration of aneurysm, and great risk of re-bleeding, short-term (72 h) therapy with tranexamic acid or aminocaproic acid is advisable (provided there is no medical contraindication) to decrease the risk of early bleeding. The overall outcome did not noticeably improve in patients treated with tranexamic acid, in spite of a remarkable decrease in re-bleeding [3, 6].

In an uncontrolled study of 18 patients who received an intraoperative dose of Recombinant factor VIIa, no re-bleeding was reported; however, one case had deep venous thrombosis (DVT) and seven had thrombosis in upper extremity in association with peripherally inserted central lines. Currently, there is no evidence to support the use of recombinant factor VIIa [3].

9.1.2. Vasospasm

Vasospasm is luminal narrowing of large cerebral blood arteries after SAH, leading to cerebral ischemia. Vasospasm commonly occurs 3–5 days after initial hemorrhage, with peak vasoconstriction occurring between days 5 and 14; it usually resolves spontaneously after 21 days of SAH. It may manifest in many features such as reduced conscious level, focal neurological deficit, and simply nuchal rigidity; the exclusion of other causes, such as re-bleeding, hydrocephalus, sepsis, and metabolic derangement, is required to confirm the diagnosis [6, 14, 15].

Sometimes there is no correlation between severity of vasospasm and the symptoms of ischemia. There are patients with severe large artery spasm who never become symptomatic and others with quite modest spasm who develop infarction. Possibly various factors play important role in the development of ischemia and infarction, such as distal microcirculatory failure, poor collateral anatomy, and genetic or physiological variations in cellular ischemic tolerance. Vasospasm is confirmed angiographically in 70% of SAH patient, however it manifests as symptomatic spasm in 36% of all patients with SAH [6, 14, 15].

Age more than 80 years, smoking, hypertension, SAH clot volume (a higher Fisher's grade), location of aneurysm (vertebral artery, right sylvian fissure, pericallosal middle cerebral artery [MCA]), left ventricular hypertrophy, and treatment modality are the main risk factors for the development of cerebral vasospasm [15].

Digital subtraction angiography (DSA) is the gold standard diagnostic investigation to diagnose vasospasm (reduced arterial diameter). Computed tomography angiography (CTA) and MRI studies are alternative investigations to DSA [15].

Transcranial Doppler sonography (TCD) can be used at the bedside to aid the diagnosis of vasospasm. The TCD criteria for vasospasm include a mean flow velocity (MFV) greater than 120 cm/s, change in MFV value of more than 50 cm/s over 24 h, and Lindegaard ratio more than 3 (Lindegaard is a ratio derived from concurrent measurements of MFV in MCA and distal ipsilateral extracranial ICA). Diffusion-perfusion mismatch on MRI is an useful investigation for the identification of early stages of vasospasm. Increase in motor-evoked potential threshold more than 50 mA from the baseline value is an accurate indicator of vasospasm.

Inflammatory marker such as C-reactive protein has been investigated for its ability to predict vasospasm. In 93 SAH patients, postoperative and not preoperative C-reactive proteins were associated with vasospasm and poor outcome with a cut-off value of 4 mg/dL [15].

9.1.2.1. Pathophysiology of cerebral vasospasm

It is complicated. Various cascades in affected blood vessels and neurons are in play, they can be grouped into two categories.

9.1.2.1.1. Elevated intracellular calcium

After SAH, calcium influxes into smooth muscle and neuron is rapidly increased through N-methyl-D-aspartate receptor (NMDA) and voltage-gated calcium channels, moreover glutamate is increased and activates NMDA receptors, leading to further calcium influx in smooth muscle, high intracellular calcium concentration enhances binding of calcium to calmodulin. Calmodulin activates myosin light chain kinase (MLCK) to phosphorylate myosin, which induces myosin-actin interaction and smooth muscle contraction and blood vessels constriction [14].

In neuronal cells, increase in intracellular calcium leads to hyperactivation of enzymes, such as protease, endonuclease, phospholipase, which destabilizes cell body and membrane, leading to cellular injury and death [14].

9.1.2.1.2. Vasoactive compound and vessel wall injury

In days 3–5 after SAH, oxy hemoglobin—a red blood cell breakdown product—inhibits nitric oxide (physiologic vasodilator) and stimulates leukocytes to produce endothelin-1 (physiologic vasoconstrictor), resulting in potent vasoconstriction. Furthermore, breakdown of oxyhemoglobin leads to release of reactive oxygen species and iron which leads to oxidative damage to blood vessel walls [14].

In addition, production of vasoactive compounds after SAH, such as serotonin, norepinephrine, and angiotensin II, leads to potent vasoconstriction [14].

9.1.2.2. Treatment of cerebral vasospasm and cerebral ischemia

9.1.2.2.1. Nimodipine

It is L-type calcium channel blocker—it is the only drug that has been approved for SAH in European countries and the USA. It improves long-term neurological outcome if it is started on admission and administered for 21 days. The recommended oral dosage is 60 mg 4 hourly orally (maximum daily dose 360 mg). The role of nimodipine is based on general brain protective mechanism as there is no proof to suggest that it treats angiographically diagnosed vasospasm, and it also increases fibrinolytic activity and inhibits cortical spreading ischemia [2, 6, 12, 15].

Recently, biodegradable silica-based nimodipine implant was effectively used in the management of vasospasm. It is associated with higher nimodipine cerebrospinal fluid (CSF) to plasma ratio than traditional nimodipine [15].

The continuous intravenous infusion of nimodipine is not recommended as it is not superior to oral nimodipine and is associated with high incidence of hypotension especially in hypovolemic patient (an adequate systolic BP of 130–150 mmHg takes priority over nimodipine administration, and it should be stopped if a stable BP can't be maintained).

The recommended dose of Intravenous nimodipine is 1 mg/h in the first 6 h, then increased to 1.5 mg/h in next 6 h, then increased to 2 mg/h (maximum dose) [2, 6, 15].

9.1.2.2.2. Fasudil

It is Rho-kinase inhibitor, it decreases smooth muscle contraction and inhibits TNF-induced IL-6 release from C6 glioma cells, and it causes better angiographic reduction in vasospasm and better neurological outcome than nimodipine. Fasudil is approved for use in Japan and China but not in the USA or Europe [12, 15].

9.1.2.2.3. Triple-H therapy (hemodynamic augmentation therapy)

It is a combination of induced hypertension, hypervolemia, and hemodilution (HHH) to improve blood flow through narrowed cerebral blood vessels due to vasospasm. Triple-H has been for years used as a treatment of choice for the treatment of delayed cerebral ischemia, although the literature supporting its effectiveness and safety is lacking, in fact triple-H therapy is associated with an increase in the risk of systemic complications such as heart failure, pulmonary edema, and infections; therefore, the use of prophylactic triple-H therapy is not recommended [3, 12].

Angiographic vasospasm without a new neurological deficit should not be treated. The development of unexplained new neurological deficit or change in conscious level, immediate aggressive therapy should be started. The first step is a fluid bolus with normal saline to increase cerebral blood flow (CBF) in ischemic area, the goal is to maintain euvolemia. Hypervolemia and hemodilution do not increase cerebral oxygen delivery and might cause adverse events. If patients fail to respond completely to the fluid, management may undergo a trial of hypertension. Blood pressure is increased gradually with the use of a vasopressor. Neurological assessment should be repeated frequently in each blood pressure step (systolic blood pressure 180 mmHg / 190 mmHg / 200 mmHg), and the target should be based on neurological improvement. If the patient did not respond to induced hypertension (systolic blood pressure of 200–220 mmHg), a rescue cerebral angioplasty should be considered [12].

9.1.2.2.4. Balloon angioplasty

Cerebral angioplasty is indicated in symptomatic patient with cerebral vasospasm, who is not responding to hypertensive therapy, Prophylactic angioplasty is not recommended [2, 6, 12].

Cerebral angioplasty may lead to arterial dissection, rupture, thrombosis, infarction, hemorrhage, and reperfusion injury leading to cerebral edema [6, 15].

9.1.2.2.5. Intra-arterial papaverine

Up to 300 mg of papaverine per hemisphere is used for the treatment of distal vasospasm.

The main disadvantages of intra-arterial papaverine may require repeating, relatively short-acting, neurotoxic, seizures, blindness, coma, irreversible brain injury, arrhythmia, and hemodynamic instability refractory to treatment [2].

9.1.2.2.6. Magnesium sulphate

Currently, there is no evidence to support the use of magnesium sulphate ($MgSO_4$) prophylactically or as a treatment modality in delayed cerebral ischemia (DCI). In the Mash 2 Trial, $MgSO_4$ did not improve primary outcome. However, intrathecal and cisternal administration of $MgSO_4$ significantly decreased the severity of vasospasm without any reduction in incidence of DCI or functional outcome [3, 6, 15].

9.1.2.2.7. Statins

Recent meta-analysis reported no role of statin in SAH, and a larger phase 3 trial (Simvastatin in Aneurysmal Subarachnoid Hemorrhage [STASH]) failed to confirm any beneficial effect of statin for long- or short-term outcome and should not be used routinely in acute stage [6, 12, 15].

9.1.2.2.8. Endothelin A-receptor antagonist

Clazosentan (endothelin-1 receptor antagonist) had been presented to be associated with a dose-dependent decrease in the frequency of vasospasm in a phase IIb trial (Clazosentan to Overcome Neurological iSChemia and Infarct OccUrring after Subarachnoid hemorrhage [CONSCIOUS-1]) [6, 15].

Two further trials were carried out:

CONSCIOUS-2: A double blind, placebo-controlled trial, clazosentan was given at a rate of 5 mg/h for 15 days to patients treated with aneurysm clipping. There was statistically insignificant decrease in mortality and vasospasm-related morbidity [15].

CONSCIOUS-3: This study was double blind, placebo- controlled study to assess whether clazosentan reduced vasospasm-related mortality after securing aneurysmal SAH by endovascular coiling. The study was halted prematurely after completion of conscious-2 trial and failed to show any beneficial effect of clazosentan.

It is worth noting that patient who received clazosentan had more pulmonary complications, anemia, and hypotension than the placebo group [6, 15].

9.1.2.3. Other miscellaneous treatments

9.1.2.3.1. Milrinone

In a large case series based on the assessment of all subarachnoid hemorrhage patients diagnosed with delayed ischemic neurological deficit between April 1999 and April 2006, 88 patients were found to have received milrinone infusion for a median of 9.8 days. At 44.6 months, 75% of them had a good functional outcome. Because of obvious limitations in this study, further studies are warranted [15].

9.1.2.3.2. Stellate ganglion block

A small study included 15 patients who had refractory cerebral vasospasm after surgical clipping of aneurysm. Stellate ganglion block was performed using 10 mL of bupivacaine 0.5% on the side with maximum cerebral blood flow velocity. Neurological status, cerebral blood flow velocity, and pulsatility index were assessed before and 10 min, 30 min, 2 h, 6 h, 12 h, and 24 h after stellate ganglion block. The ipsilateral Middle Cerebral Artery (MCA) mean velocity was reduced with reduction in neurological deficit and improvement in GCS; because of obvious limitations in this study, further studies are required [15].

9.1.2.3.3. Albumin

Albumin 25% has been tried to improve outcomes in a pilot study (Albumin in Subarachnoid Hemorrhage trial). The incidence of vasospasm, DCI, and cerebral infarction was significantly reduced with high dose of albumin; however, this is still experimental and further studies are required to support this study [12, 15].

9.1.3. Hydrocephalus

Hydrocephalus is one of the common complications of SAH; it is either acute or chronic.

Acute hydrocephalus occurs in 15–87% of SAH patients as a result of obstruction of CSF flow by blood products or adhesion, some clinician avoid insertion of a ventricular drain in these cases immediately as half of them will recover spontaneously and there is a risk of re-bleeding and infection (meningitis and ventriculitis). Another approach recommended is to start immediate external ventricular drainage (keeping intracranial pressure between 10 and 20 mm Hg), especially when obstructive hydrocephalus is suspected or when the lumbar drainage is contraindicated (sever high intracranial pressure) [3, 6].

It has been recommended to apply lumbar drainage as a consecutive treatment of external ventricular drain (EVD) before shunting in cases with spontaneous intracerebral hemorrhage (ICH) when there is no blood in the third and fourth ventricles (communicating hydrocephalus). This option can be considered as an alternate approach to decrease the occurrence of permanent shunts, improve brain relaxation, and decrease risk of vasospasm; however, this approach may cause downward herniation in some cases such as supratentorial swelling and the development of hygroma. Currently no prospective clinical trial supports lumbar drain insertion either for spontaneous ICH or cases with SAH [3, 6].

Acute hydrocephalus increases risk of cerebral infarction and re-bleeding and eventually may worsen the mortality and morbidity secondary to cerebral infarction and re-bleeding [3, 6].

Chronic shunt-dependent hydrocephalus, which occurs in 8.9–48% of patients with SAH due to a decrease in CSF absorption at the arachnoid granulation, it is usually treated with shunt placement [3, 6].

Many factors are considered as predictor of hydrocephalus:

- Elderly.

- Intraventricular hemorrhage.

- Hypertension.

- Hyponatremia at presentation.

- Low Glasgow Coma Score at presentation.

- Antifibrinolytic agents.

9.1.4. Seizures

More than 26% of patients with SAH experience seizure-like episodes, the majority of such patients report the onset of these seizures occurring before medical care are accessed. There are variable risk factors for the development of early seizures, such as aneurysm in middle cerebral artery, thickness of SAH clot, hypertension, intracerebral hematoma, re-bleeding, cerebral infarction, and poor neurological grade. Routine use of anticonvulsants is associated with worsening of the cognitive function, delayed ischemia, fever, and vasospasm; however, it may be considered in patients with high risk of delayed seizure [3, 6].

9.2. Systemic complications associated with SAH

The high morbidity and mortality associated with SAH is not only due to neurological complications, non-neurological complications also play a major role in increasing mortality and morbidity rates [16].

9.2.1. Cardiac complications

Cardiac complications occur in about 50% of patients with SAH; it ranges from mild elevation in cardiac enzymes and electrocardiogram (ECG) changes to obvious clinical and echocardiographic pathology. Cardiac damage markers are associated with an increased mortality and poor outcome and DCI [16].

9.2.1.1. Pathophysiology

9.2.1.1.1. Mild myocardial injury

This is presented by mild elevation in serum cardiac troponin I (not reaching diagnostic threshold of MI). This elevation occurs in 20–68% of patients with SAH. The degree of neurological injury, as graded by the Hunt-Hess scale, is an independent predictor of myocardial injury in SAH patients. Serum troponin is a powerful predictor for cardiac and pulmonary complications, such as hypotension requiring vasopressor, left ventricular (LV) dysfunction, pulmonary edema, and DCI, especially in patient presenting with a high grade on WFNS.

Serum troponin is a more specific and sensitive indicator of myocardial injury than creatinine kinase-MB; therefore, serum troponin levels and trends must be monitored through serial measurements particularly in SAH patients with past history of cardiovascular disease [16].

9.2.1.1.2. Cardiomyopathy

Neurogenic stunned myocardium (NSM) is the most severe form of myocardial injury in SAH, it occurs in 20–30% of patients with SAH. The elevated level of sympathetic tone leads to calcium overload with reduced sensitization of contractile filaments to this cation, eventually causing myocardial depression. It is characterized by subendocardial contraction band necrosis.

Echocardiography shows abnormal LV contractility and abnormal wall motion, which are reversible but sometimes leads to cardiogenic shock [16].

CK-MB levels, female gender, and poor neurological grade are predictors of LV dysfunction.

Severe LV dysfunction decreases cardiac output (CO) and mean arterial pressure leading to reduction in cerebral blood flow (CBF). Furthermore, LV dysfunction may be associated with cerebral vasospasm and significant decrease in cerebral perfusion pressure therefore, optimization of heart function is critical to prevent progression of neurological dysfunction and to promote recovery in patients with SAH [2, 6, 16–18].

The use of inotropes such as dobutamine or milrinone may be required to optimize cardiac output (CO). In severe LV dysfunction, implementation of intra-aortic balloon pump may be required [2, 6, 16, 18].

9.2.1.1.3. ECG findings

It is common in SAH patients, particularly in the first 3 days of presentation, nearly 50–100% of SAH patients will show different forms of ECG changes such as ST segments changes, T wave changes, QTc prolongation, and Prominent U wave (**Table 6**) [16, 17].

Around 4–8% of SAH patients will have malignant arrhythmias such as ventricular tachycardia (VT), torsade de pointe, and asystole [16, 18].

ECG abnormality	Reported incidence (%)
ST-segment changes	15–51
Inverted or isoelectric T waves	12–92
QTc prolongation	11–66
Prominent U waves	4–47
Sinus bradycardia	16
Sinus tachycardia	8.5

Table 6. ECG changes after subarachnoid hemorrhage [17].

Management of arrhythmias in SAH patients depends upon the type of arrhythmia, clinical significance, and the patient's condition. As a first step, it is vital to assure satisfactory oxygenation and correct electrolyte abnormalities and metabolic disturbance.

The use of beta-blockers to treat cardiac tachyarrhythmia in SAH should be balanced against hypotension and decrease in cerebral blood flow (CBF). A new study concluded that the presence of arrhythmias is associated with poor outcome; in spite of this, no correlation was found between severity of cardiac arrhythmia and the site or the extent of intracranial hemorrhage on CT scan, neurological condition, or the location of ruptured malformation [6, 16, 18].

9.2.2. Electrolyte disturbance

The SAH is associated with different forms of electrolyte disturbances, such as hyponatremia, hypokalemia, hypocalcaemia, and hypomagnesaemia [6].

9.2.2.1. Hyponatremia

Hyponatremia is the most common clinically significant electrolyte derangement associated with SAH. It has an incidence ranging from 35 to 56 %, its diagnostic and therapeutic dilemma needs to be sorted to improve outcome of SAH patient [2, 16, 19].

Syndrome of inappropriate antidiuretic hormone secretion (SIADH) is the most common cause of hyponatremia; other causes are acute cortisol insufficiency, cerebral salt wasting syndrome (CSW), extreme fluid therapy, and/or diuretic therapy.

Kao et al. stated that 34.5% of severe hyponatremia were secondary to SIADH, whereas 23% were considered to be due to CSW. Noteworthy, the patients recruited in this study had more severe SAH than in the comparative studies, and the inclusion criterion was a plasma Na <130 mEq/L [19].

Irrespective of the cause, hyponatremia in SAH patients increases hospital stay, risk of vasospasm, and mortality rate.

The incidence of hyponatremia is associated with the location of aneurysmal rupture. Hyponatremia mostly occurs after rupture of anterior communicating artery (AComA). It was seen in 52.4% of patients with AComA; it may be because the hypothalamus is supplied by branch from AComA [19].

9.2.2.2. Causes of hyponatremia

SIADH is considered the most common cause of severe hyponatremia in SAH; it is secondary to excessive secretion of antidiuretic hormone as a result of stimulation of hypothalamus with traumatic or ischemic factor, causing increased water reabsorption in the distal convoluted tubule of the kidney, resulting in dilutional hyponatremia and fluid retention [19].

In CSW, the increase in urinary sodium excretion and urine output are due to abnormal release of atrial and brain natriuretic hormones, causing reduction in circulating blood volume, as well as extracellular fluid. Cerebral salt wasting syndrome can be treated with hypertonic saline solution which increases cerebral blood flow, brain tissue oxygen [19].

Clinically, it is very difficult to differentiate between SIADH and CSW syndrome, due to significant overlapping clinical findings between both syndromes: both syndromes are associated with brain lesions; have normal thyroid, adrenal, and kidney functions are hyponatremic, hypouricemic and have concentrated urines, high urinary sodium over 40 mEq/L, and high fractional excretion (FE) of urate. The only clinical difference is the state of their extracellular volume (ECV): being hypervolemic or euvolemic in SIADH and hypovolemic in CSW (**Table 7**) [20].

ECV assessment by usual clinical criteria is very difficult, not accurate to any degree [20].

Determination fractional excretion (FE) of urate is very helpful to differentiate between these syndromes, FEurate, normal 4–11%, has been constantly increased to >11% in both syndromes and has a distinctive relationship to serum sodium in both syndromes. In SIADH, correction of hyponatremia will normalize FEurate to 4–11% but in CSW syndrome FEurate consistently > 11% event after correction of hyponatremia (**Figure 3**).

This algorithm is useful only with normal glomerular filtration rate GFR, because FEurate can exceed normal values in patients with reduced glomerular filtration rate (GFR) [20].

Cortisol deficiency is one of the important causes of hyponatremia, which has not been well investigated in SAH patients because routine examination of adrenocorticotropic hormone (ACTH)/cortisol dynamic is not part of SAH work up [19].

Klose et al. and Parenti et al. investigated pituitary function post-SAH and found that between 7.1 and 12% of patients are cortisol-deficient at the time of presentation with SAH [20].

	SIADH	CSW
Plasma volume	↑ or ↔	↓↓
Water balance	↑ or ↔	Negative
Signs and symptoms of dehydration	Absent	Present
Central venous pressure	↑ or ↔	↓↓
Salt balance	Variable	Negative
Hematocrit	↔	↑ or ↔
Serum osmolality	↓↓	↓↓
Urine sodium	↑	↑↑
Urine volume	↓ or ↔	↑↑
Plasma BUN/creatinine	↓↓	↑ or ↔
Treatment	Fluid restriction, hypertonic saline, furosemide, demeclocycline	Normal saline, hypertonic saline, fludrocortisone

Table 7. Difference between SIADH and CSW [21].

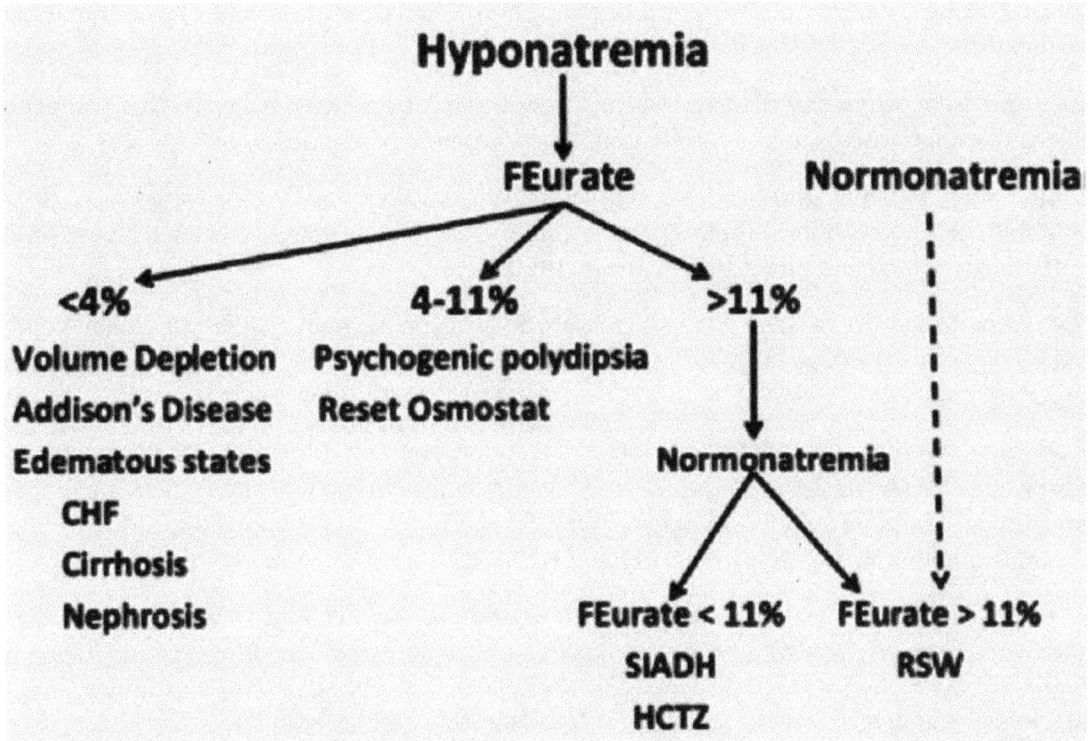

Figure 3. Algorithm for determining the cause of hyponatremia, using FEurate.

9.2.2.3. Treatment of hyponatremia

Patients with SAH should be closely monitored in an intensive care unit, preferably neurointensive care for at least 2–3 weeks post-SAH, to allow for close monitoring of signs and symptoms of delayed cerebral ischemia (DCI), cerebral vasospasm, as well as fluid and electrolyte balance on daily basis, which can help treating doctors in early detection and efficient management of hyponatremia. A daily follow-up of electrolyte is ideal and should be routine. If patients require intravenous hypertonic saline, sodium level should be checked every 4 h.

Urgent investigations of sodium level are mandatory if there are changes in mental status, massive fluctuation of fluid balance, and/or polyuria.

Rapid correction of hyponatremia can cause central myelinolysis and should be avoided, but insufficient correction of hyponatremia can result in brain edema, convulsion, and death [17, 20–22].

Fluid restriction to correct hyponatremia is associated with increased risk of cerebral vasospasm [19, 23].

Audibert et al. looked at the endocrinological response to severe SAH and found alterations in plasma level of numerous hormones such as aldosterone, renin, ADH, angiotensin, ANP, and BNP. However, these changes are noted during the first 12 days post-SAH. It is not practical to correctly and promptly get hormone levels, because their profile fluctuates frequently.

The expertise recommended that assessing bedside sodium and fluid balance is the best valuable and economical technique for avoiding hyponatremia in patients with SAH [17].

Traditionally, patients with SAH are maintained on sodium chloride-based fluids (i.e., 0.9% saline) for baseline and fluid replacement requirements, to avoid cerebral edema due to fluid shifts across a damaged blood-brain barrier [19].

The recent guidelines of the Neurocritical Care Society for the management of patients with SAH suggested avoiding large amounts of free water intake and fluid restriction to treat hyponatremia [19].

In addition, the guidelines of the American Heart Association recommend that volume contraction be replaced with isotonic fluids (Class IIa, Level B evidence) and that large volumes of hypotonic fluids should be avoided in patients with SAH. The guidelines, however, did not make recommendations on the composition of baseline fluid administration in SAH patients [17].

Recently, Lehmann et al. suggested balanced crystalloids and colloid solutions (those with electrolyte compositions similar to plasma) in SAH patients, which do not cause frequent hyponatremia or hypo-osmolality, also prevent electrolyte imbalance such as hyperchloremia, hyper osmolality, and extreme positive fluid balances associated with saline-based intravenous fluids [19, 24].

Fluid restriction to less than 500 mL/day is the treatment of choice in SIADH, although such approach may not be feasible in SAH, because fluid restriction can cause cerebral vasospasm and subsequently cerebral infarction. What's more, most of these patients are not fully conscious and require enteral feeding which results in a daily fluid intake of 1–2 L [19, 25].

Therapeutic options for water restriction include hypertonic saline solutions and albumin [19]. Hypertonic saline (2–3% solution) not only increases plasma sodium concentration efficiently and rapidly but also increases the risk of pulmonary edema and heart failure and neurological complications secondary to the increase in blood volume [19].

Fludrocortisone causes sodium retention, but it is associated with fluid overload and limited evidence of its effectiveness [19].

Vasopressin receptor antagonists such as conivaptan have been projected and trialed in small studies but have not become routine therapy, because harmful effect secondary to the rapid increase in plasma sodium (4–6 mEq/L) [19, 26].

Acute cortisol deficiency is typically corrected with administration of parenteral hydrocortisone, but the beneficial effect of hydrocortisone is still uncertain and further studies are required, because it is not clear whether corticosteroid therapy is effective in management of acute relative adrenal insufficiency after SAH [19, 27].

Overall, the management of hyponatremia in SAH patients necessitates additional investigation of treatment options that avoid fluid restriction, and further studies will help standardize ideal care.

9.2.3. Fever

Fever is one of the common medical complications of SAH and occurs in 70% of SAH patients. Fever may be due hypothalamic effect of the hemorrhage; it is associated with the severity of the injury, amount of hemorrhage, and development of vasospasm. Effective fever management may improve functional outcome. Paracetamol is the treatment of choice for fever. Active cooling is very effective but adverse effects of shivering may offset its benefit [6, 17].

It is worth noting that the infectious cause such as pneumonia needs to be excluded [17].

9.2.4. Anemia

Anemia is very common and is associated with poor outcome, due to compromising brain oxygen delivery. Correction of anemia and high hemoglobin value improve outcome after SAH. Current guidance recommends to keep hemoglobin concentration between 8 and 10 g/dL [17].

9.2.5. Thrombocytopenia and deep venous thrombosis (DVT)

Heparin-induced thrombocytopenia (HIT) is directly associated with the number of angiographic procedures have been performed. Patients with heparin-induced thrombocytopenia type II seems to be at high risk of thrombotic complications, vasospasm, and poor outcome.

Currently, it is uncertain whether there is practical means of avoiding HIT (as it is essential in angiographic procedures); however, it is vital to know this complication to avoid further heparin exposure and to use non-heparin substitute under the supervision of a hematologist.

DVT is relatively recurrent event after SAH, especially in immobilized patients [3, 6].

Table 8 and **Figure 4** summarize the incidence rate of non-neurological complications.

Complications	Incidence (%)
Fever	54
Anemia	36
Hyperglycemia	30
Hypertension	27
Hypernatremia	22
Pneumonia	20
Hypotension	18
Pulmonary edema	14
Hyponatremia	14
Life-threatening arrhythmia	8
Myocardial ischemia	6

Table 8. Non-neurological complications of subarachnoid hemorrhage [17].

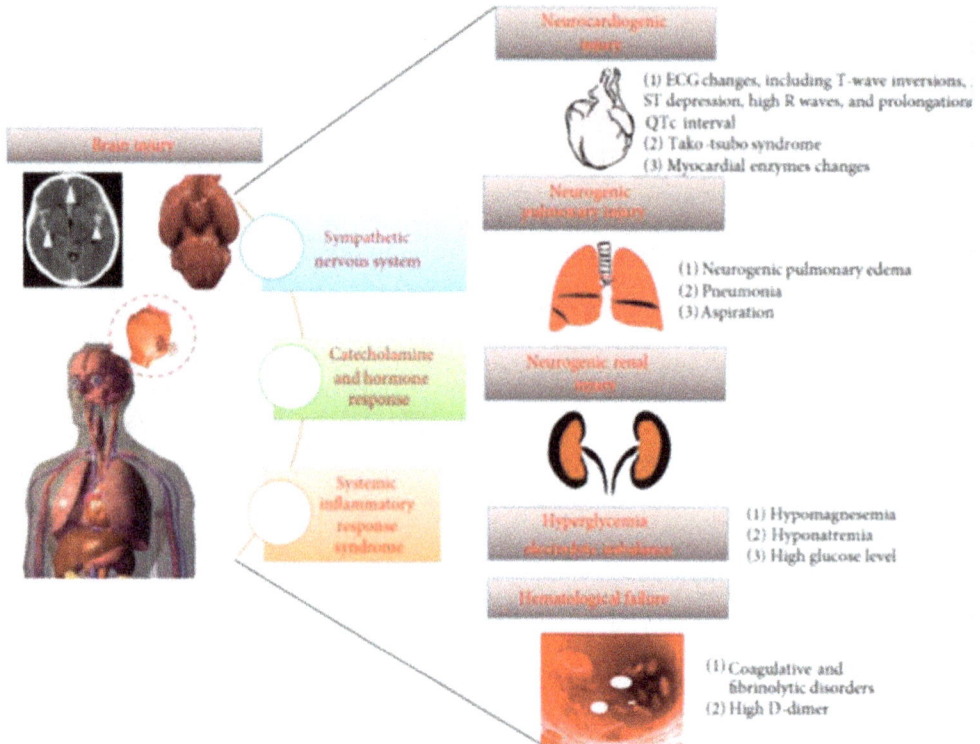

Figure 4. Harmful effects of SAH on extracerebral organs [28].

10. Surgical and endovascular methods for treatment of ruptured cerebral aneurysms

Ruptured aneurysms can be cured by microsurgical clipping or endovascular coiling.

Microsurgical clipping requires craniotomy to prevent re-bleeding of the aneurysm via insertion of a clip through its neck, thus isolating the aneurysm from circulation. This technique conveys a 98% certainty of elimination of the risk of rupture [29].

Endovascular coiling is the blocking of an aneurysm by an endovascular approach with electrically detachable platinum coils device which induces secondary thrombosis of the aneurysm [6]. The first published prospective randomized outcome study of surgical versus endovascular coiling, concluded that endovascular treatment results in clinical outcomes equal to that of surgical clipping.

Koivisto and co-worker (2000) published first prospective randomized outcome study of surgical versus endovascular coiling, they concluded that endovascular treatment results in clinical outcomes equal to that of surgical clipping [30].

The International Subarachnoid Aneurysm Trial (ISAT) is the first multicenter prospective randomized trial comparing the two options; the included 2143 patients with ruptured intracranial aneurysms were randomly assigned to clipping (1070) or coiling (1073). Primary outcomes included death or dependent living, and secondary outcomes included risk of seizures and risk of re-bleeding. Initially, 1-year outcomes concluded a fall in death and disability from 31% in the clipping arm to 24% in the endovascular arm, this difference was mainly driven by a reduction in the rate of disability among survivors (16% in the endovascular arm and 22% in the clipping arm) [6, 29, 30].

The risk of epilepsy and significant cognitive decline was also reduced in the endovascular group, but the occurrence of late re-bleeding was increased in endovascular group (2.9% after endovascular repair vs. 0.9% after open surgery) and only 58% of coiled aneurysms were completely obliterated compared with 81% of clipped aneurysms [6].

Although these results have affected the approach to patients with intracranial aneurysm in neurosurgical centers across the world, the study has been criticized due to the lack of generalizability, for example, posterior circulation aneurysms, which account for 8% of patients admitted with subarachnoid hemorrhage and up to 48% of ruptured aneurysms managed by endovascular coiling at some centers, made up only 2.7% of the ISAT study population [30].

Tahir et al. [29] concluded no significant difference in the clinical outcome of coiling and clipping of ruptured intracranial aneurysms; however, clipping is more cost effective than coiling.

Clipping is recommended for middle cerebral artery aneurysms (difficult to treat with endovascular technique) and patients presenting with an intraparenchymal hematoma >50 mL (high occurrence of critical outcome). Endovascular coiling is the preferred technique for patients presenting with vasospasm, elderly, poor clinical grade, and posterior cerebral aneurysms [6].

11. Time of surgical intervention

The most important strategy to reduce the risk of aneurysm rupture is early aneurysm repair, although evidence for best time of intervention is limited, it is uncertain whether ultra- early treatment (before 24 h) is better than aneurysm repair within 72 h (early). Recently published data analysis suggested that the surgical intervention can be done safely within 72 h after SAH. The American Heart Association/American Stroke Association recommend that "surgical clipping or endovascular coiling of the ruptured aneurysm should be performed as early as feasible in the majority of patients to reduce the rate of re-bleeding after SAH" (Class 1B). This recommendation is supported by the European Stroke Organization Guidelines for the Management of Intracranial Aneurysms and Subarachnoid Haemorrhage, which indicated that "aneurysm should be treated as early as logistically and technically possible to reduce the risk of re-bleeding; if possible it should be aimed to intervene at least within 72 hours after onset of first symptoms." There is ongoing study that only recruiting SAH with poor grade may help answer the question of whether intervention within 72 h (early intervention) is associated with better outcome compared with intervention within 4–7 days [12].

12. Prognosis and outcome

In spite of improvement in interventional and medical treatment of SAH, rupture of an aneurysm is still associated with significant high mortality rates (about 33%) and sever disability

(17%). In last decades, mortality rates decreased by 17%, and the chance to recover to independent state has increased by 1.5% per year. Severity of initial bleeding plays a vital role in the determination of mortality rate and functional outcome [3].

Age is another important factor: mortality rate increased three times if the patient was older than 80 years. Aneurysm size, site, history of hypertension, high systolic pressure, history of alcohol consumption, cigarette smoking are all important factors associated with poor outcome regardless the severity of SAH [3].

Complications such as re-bleeding, DCI, hydrocephalus, hyperglycemia, metabolic disturbances, cardiopulmonary complications, prolonged bed rest are associated with increased probability of poor outcome.

Small studies suggest that increased catecholamine levels in cerebrospinal fluid (CSF) are associated with early mortality or disability. Serum S100 is another marker of poor outcome after SAH [3].

13. Conclusion

Aneurysmal SAH is a devastating neurovascular disease associated with very high mortality and morbidity despite improvement in interventional and medical treatment due to multiple neurological and systemic complications, especially re-bleeding and DCI secondary to vasospasm. Age, smoking, alcohol consumption, hypertension, site and size of aneurysm are important factors associated with poor outcome. SAH needs multidisciplinary specialized care, best provided in high-volume centers to improve outcome.

Author details

Adel E. Ahmed Ganaw*, Abdulgafoor M. Tharayil, Ali O. Mohamed Bel Khair, Saher Tahseen, Jazib Hassan, Mohammad Faisal Abdullah Malmstrom and Sohel Mohamed Gamal Ahmed

*Address all correspondence to: adelganaw@yahoo.co.uk

Department of Anesthesiology, ICU and Perioperative Medicine, Hamad Medical Corporation, Doha, Qatar

References

[1] Vlak MH, Algra A, Brandenburg R, Rinkel GJ. Prevalence of unruptured intracranial aneurysms, with emphasis on sex, age, comorbidity, country, and time period: A systematic review and meta-analysis. Lancet Neurology. 2011;**10**:626

[2] Daniel C. Subarachnoid hemorrhage disease and anaesthetist. South African Journal of Anaesthesia and Analgesia. Vol 16 no 1(2010); 60-68

[3] Steiner T, Juvela S, Unterberg A, Jung C. European stroke organization guidelines for the management of intracranial aneurysms and subarachnoid haemorrhage. Cerebrovascular Diseases. 2013;**35**:93-112. DOI: 10.1159/000346087

[4] Kothandaraman U, Lokanadham S. Review on anatomy of cerebral arterial system—Clinical importance. Journal of Clinical and Biomedical Sciences. 2014;**4**(3):305-308

[5] Moss C, Wilson SR. Subarachnoid haemorrhage and anaesthesia for neurovascular surgery. Anesthesia and Intensive Care Medicine. 2011; 204-207.

[6] Sander Connolly E, Jr, Rabinstein Alejandro A, Ricardo Carhuapoma J, Derdeyn Colin P, Jacques D, Higashida Randall T, et al. Guidelines for the management of aneurysmal subarachnoid hemorrhage: Guidelines for healthcare professionals from the American heart association/American stroke association. Stroke. 2012;**43**:1711-1737

[7] Aoki T, Kataoka H, Shimamura M, Nakagami H, Wakayama K, Moriwaki T, et al. NF-κB is a key mediator of cerebral aneurysm formation. Circulation. 2007;**116**:2830-2840

[8] Evans RW, Dilli E, Dodick DW. Sentinel headache. Headache. 2009;**49**:599-603

[9] Czuczman AD, Thomas LE, Boulanger AB, Peak DA, Senecal EL, Brown DF, Marill KA. Interpreting red blood cells in lumbar puncture: Distinguishing true subarachnoid hemorrhage from traumatic tap. Academic Emergency Medicine. 2013;**20**:247

[10] Rosen DS, Macdonald LR. Subarachnoid hemorrhage grading scales. Neurocritical Care. 2005;**2**:110-118. DOI: 10.1385/

[11] Fernández TT, Capilla ME, *Morcillo CR*, Gonzalez RGG, Herrera I, Benassi GJM. Vasospasm After Subarachnoid Hemorrhage: Utility of Perfusion CT and CT Angiography on Diagnosis of Delayed Cerebral Ischemia. Spain: Department of Neuroradiology at Virgen de la Salud Hospital Toledo. ECR 2016/C-0298

[12] de Oliveira Manoel AL, Goffi A, Marotta TR, Schweizer TA, Abrahamson S, Macdonald LR. The critical care management of poorgrade subarachnoid haemorrhage. Critical Care. 2016;**20**:21. DOI: 10.1186/s13054-016-1193-9

[13] Naidech AM, Janjua N, Kreiter KT, Ostapkovich ND, Fitzsimmons BF, Parra A, et al. Predictors and impact of aneurysm rebleeding after subarachnoid hemorrhage. Archives of Neurology. 2005;**62**:410

[14] Chen T, Carter B. Role of magnesium sulphate in aneurysmal SAH management: A meta-analysis of controlled trial. Asian Journal of the Neurosurgery. 2011;**6**:1

[15] Ganne S, Rao U, Muthuchellappan R. Cerebral vasospasm: Current understanding. Current Opinion in Anesthesiology. 2016;**29**:544-551. DOI: 10.1097/ACO.0000000000000370

[16] Behrouz R, Sullebarger JT, Malek AR. Cardiac manifestations of subarachnoid hemorrhage. Expert Review of Cardiovascular Therapy. 2011;**9**(3):303307

[17] Highton D, Smith M. Intensive care management of subarachnoid haemorrhage 2C04,3C00, review article. The Intensive Care Society. 2013; 28-35

[18] Chatterjee S. ECG changes in subarachnoid haemorrhage: A synopsis. Netherlands Heart Journal. 2011;**19**:31-34. DOI: 10.1007/s12471-010-0049-1

[19] Marupudi NI, Mittal S. Diagnosis and management of hyponatremia in patients with aneurysmal subarachnoid hemorrhage. Journal of Clinical Medicine. 2015;**4**:756-767. DOI: 10.3390/jcm4040756

[20] Maesaka JK, Imbriano L, Mattana J, Gallagher D, Bade N, Sharif S. Differentiating SIADH from cerebral/renal salt wasting: Failure of the volume approach and need for a new approach to hyponatremia. Journal of Clinical Medicine. 2014;**3**:1373-1385. DOI: 10.3390/jcm3041373

[21] Cerdà-Esteve M, et al. Cerebral salt wasting syndrome. Review. European Journal of Internal Medicine. 2008;19:249-254.

[22] Gharaibeh KA, Brewer JM, Agarwal M, Fulop T. Risk factors, complication and measures to prevent or reverse catastrophic sodium overcorrection in chronic hyponatremia. American Journal of the Medical Sciences. 2015;**349**:170-175

[23] Tommasino C, Moore S, Todd MM. Cerebral effects of isovolemic hemodilution with crystalloid or colloid solutions. Critical Care Medicine. 1988;**16**: 862-868

[24] Lehmann L, Bendel S, Uehlinger DE, Takala J, Schafer M, Reinert M, Jakob SM. Randomized, double-blind trial of the effect of fluid composition on electrolyte, acid-base, and fluid homeostasis in patients early after subarachnoid hemorrhage. Neurocritical Care. 2013;**18**:5-12

[25] Bederson JB, Connolly ES, Jr, Batjer HH, Dacey RG, Dion JE, Diringer MN, et al. Guidelines for the management of aneurysmal subarachnoid hemorrhage: A statement for healthcare professionals from a special writing group of the stroke council, American heart association. Stroke. 2009;**40**:994-102

[26] Wright WL, Asbury WH, Gilmore JL, Samuels OB. Conivaptan for hyponatremia in the neurocritical care unit. Neurocritical Care. 2009;**11**:6-13

[27] Weant KA, Sasaki-Adams D, Dziedzic K, Ewend M. Acute relative adrenal insufficiency after aneurysmal subarachnoid hemorrhage. Neurosurgery. 2008;**63**:645-649

[28] Chen S, Li Q, Wu H, Krafft PR, Wang Z, Zhang JH. The harmful effects of subarachnoid hemorrhage on extracerebral organs: Review article. BioMed Research International. 2014;**2014**:12. Article ID 858496. DOI: http://dx.doi.org/10.1155/2014/858496

[29] Tahir ZM, Enam SA, Pervez AR, Bhatti A, ul Haq T. Cost-effectiveness of clipping vs. coiling of intracranial aneurysms after subarachnoid hemorrhage in a developing country. Surgical Neurology. 2009;**72**:355-361

[30] Molyneux AJ, Kerr RSC, Yu LM, Clarke M, Sneade M, Yarnold JA, Sandercock P. for the International Subarachnoid Aneurysm Trial (ISAT) Collaborative GrouISAT: Coiling or clipping for ruptured intracranial aneurysms? http://neurology.thelancet.com Vol 4 December 2005.

3

Current Perspectives on Cardiomyopathies

Nandita Mehta and Sayyidah Aasima tu Nisa Qazi

Abstract

Cardiomyopathy is a disease of the heart muscle that can affect any age group or gender and can be acquired or inherited. Its literal meaning is "heart muscle disease" and refers to the deterioration of the function of the myocardium for any reason. Cardiomyopathy affects the shape, function, and/or electrical system of the heart. Patients with cardiomyopathy can present to anaesthesiologists in emergency situations or as elective cases. The patients are usually not aware of their condition and may be diagnosed at the time of pre-anaesthetic check-up. Advanced cases are always a challenge to the anaesthesiologist as they are most commonly complicated by progressive cardiac failure. Patients with cardiomyopathy are often at risk of dysrhythmias or sudden cardiac death. This chapter describes the main features and perioperative management of patients with cardiomyopathies undergoing non-cardiac surgery. In general, the optimal anaesthetic management of patients with cardiomyopathy requires good preoperative assessment, close perioperative monitoring, suitable anaesthetic agents, optimal perioperative fluid management, and an overall stable hemodynamic status.

Keywords: anaesthesiologist, cardiomyopathy, anaesthetic management

1. Introduction

The first officially accepted definition of cardiomyopathy was given by WHO in 1980 which defined it as "heart muscle diseases of unknown cause" to differentiate cardiomyopathy from cardiac dysfunction which occurs due to known cardiovascular diseases such as hypertension, coronary artery disease, or valvular disease [1]. WHO reclassified cardiomyopathies in 1995 to include diseases of myocardium associated with cardiac dysfunction that were earlier excluded. They expanded this criterion in order to include all known causes of cardiomyopathy and is based on anatomical and physiological features. It includes three main types of cardiomyopathy: hypertrophic (HCM), dilated (DCM), and restrictive (RCM).

In 2006, American Heart Association (AHA) in their document entitled "Contemporary Definition and Classification of the Cardiomyopathies" defined cardiomyopathies as "a heterogeneous group of diseases of the myocardium associated with mechanical and/or electrical dysfunction that usually (but not invariably) exhibit inappropriate ventricular hypertrophy or dilation and are due to a variety of causes that frequently are genetic. Cardiomyopathies either are confined to the heart or are a part of generalised systemic disorders, often leading to cardiovascular death or progressive heart failure-related disability." According to the new AHA classification, cardiomyopathies are divided into two broad groups: primary cardiomyopathies and secondary cardiomyopathies. Primary cardiomyopathies encompass those that are exclusively or predominantly confined to the heart muscle and are acquired, genetic, or of mixed origin. Secondary cardiomyopathies include the subset of multiorgan involving diseases, which cause involvement of the heart as a part of their pathophysiology. In spite of this detailed classification, some confusion may arise because some primary cardiomyopathies may have associated extra cardiac components while as a few secondary cardiomyopathies can affect the heart exclusively.

Classification of primary cardiomyopathies:

Genetic	Hypertrophic cardiomyopathy
	Arrhythmogenic right ventricular cardiomyopathy
	Left ventricular noncompaction
	Glycogen storage disease
	Conduction system disease (Lenègre's disease)
	Ion channelopathies: long QT syndrome, Brugada syndrome, short QT syndrome
Mixed	Dilated cardiomyopathy
	Primary restrictive nonhypertrophied cardiomyopathy
Acquired	Myocarditis (inflammatory cardiomyopathy): viral, bacterial, rickettsial, fungal, parasitic (Chagas disease)
	Stress cardiomyopathy
	Peripartum cardiomyopathy

Classification of secondary cardiomyopathies:

Infiltrative	Amyloidosis
	Gaucher's disease
	Hunter's syndrome
Storage	Hemochromatosis
	Glycogen storage disease
	Niemann-Pick disease

Toxic	Drugs: cocaine, alcohol
	Chemotherapy drugs: doxorubicin, daunorubicin, cyclophosphamide
	Heavy metals: lead, mercury
	Radiation therapy
Inflammatory	Sarcoidosis
Endomyocardial	Hypereosinophilic (Löffler's) syndrome
	Endomyocardial fibrosis
Endocrine	Diabetes mellitus
	Hyper- or hypothyroidism
	Pheochromocytoma
	Acromegaly
Neuromuscular	Duchenne-Becker dystrophy
	Neurofibromatosis
	Tuberous sclerosis
Autoimmune	Lupus erythematosus
	Rheumatoid arthritis
	Scleroderma
	Dermatomyositis
	Polyarteritis nodosa

European Society of Cardiology in 2008 introduced a classification in which they accommodated five specific types of cardiomyopathies along with their genetic involvement: dilated, hypertrophic, arrhythmogenic, restrictive, and unclassified [2]. They further divided them into familial (genetic) or non-familial (non-genetic).

The most recent classification known as the MOGE(S) classification system had been introduced which is based on phenotype and genotype an it incorporates information on structural and functional abnormalities (M), organ involvement (O), genetics (G), aetiology (E), and disease severity (S) associated with the condition [3]. However, it cannot be considered as complete as it does not include certain cardiomyopathies like postpartum cardiomyopathy or the risk of sudden death and is very complex to use. The MOGES classification is beyond the scope of this review so we do not discuss it here.

2. Pathophysiology

Cardiomyopathy itself can present as either systolic dysfunction or diastolic dysfunction, which in turn are both related to the ventricular dysfunction.

Systolic dysfunction: This type of dysfunction is mainly seen in dilated cardiomyopathy. The predominant pathophysiology is a global decrease in myocardial contractility, which in turn leads to reduction in left ventricular ejection fraction. In the initial phases, the heart tries to compensate this change by increasing the size of left ventricular cavity which allows for an improvement in stroke volume with an associated improved force of contraction. As the disease progresses, these compensatory mechanisms prove to be inadequate in maintaining the cardiac output, eventually leading to the failure of left heart.

Diastolic dysfunction: This is the most common type of dysfunction associated with the cardiomyopathies, occurring in HCM, RCM, and other types of cardiomyopathies. The main pathophysiology is impairment of filling of blood in the left ventricle, which leads to increase in the left ventricular filling pressures. During the beginning of the diastolic phase of a normal cardiac cycle, left ventricle undergoes the phase of Isometric relaxation (which is an energy dependent process) just before the start of left ventricle filling phase. This relaxation continues in the early left ventricular filling phase. The later part of the left ventricular filling is a passive process and depends on the compliance of the left ventricle. Diastolic dysfunction can be because of the impairment of any of the two phases: active relaxation or left ventricular compliance or a combination of the two. Ischaemia mainly affects the phase of isometric relaxation, while intrinsic myocardial pathologies including fibrosis or external restriction due to pericardial diseases may lead to a reduction in left ventricular compliance.

The main types of cardiomyopathy that we come across clinically in our day-to-day practice are:

- Dilated cardiomyopathy
- Hypertrophic cardiomyopathy
- Restrictive cardiomyopathy
- Arrhythmogenic right ventricular dysplasia
- Peripartum cardiomyopathy

Some other types of cardiomyopathy are known as "unclassified cardiomyopathy." Another type of cardiomyopathy known as Takotsubo cardiomyopathy has been recently listed and is also known as "stress-induced cardiomyopathy," or broken heart syndrome.

Therefore, we focus our attention towards the commonest types of cardiomyopathies in this chapter.

3. Dilated cardiomyopathy

Dilated cardiomyopathy (DCM) is defined by cardiac enlargement with impaired systolic function of one or both ventricles. It is defined by the presence of:

a. Fractional myocardial shortening <25% and/or ejection fraction <45%.

b. Left ventricular end-diastolic diameter > 117% excluding any known cause of myocardial disease.

Familial DCM contribute about 20–48% of all DCM and can defined by

- the presence of two or more affected relatives with DCM meeting the above criteria or

- a relative of a DCM patient with unexplained sudden death before the age of 35.

The prevalence of DCM is 920/100,000 individuals and is common in Afro-Caribbean population. It is the commonest form of cardiomyopathy and is the third most common cause of congestive heart failure. DCM is the commonest indication for heart transplantation. In 30–40% patients, it is transmitted in an autosomal dominant fashion while in others it can be post viral or idiopathic. It can be of ischemic or nonischemic variety with ischemic type being related to atherosclerosis or CAD. The nonischemic variety may present itself secondary to the use of chemotherapeutic agents (doxorubicin and adriamycin), infections (Coxsackie virus, HIV, cytomegalovirus Chagas' disease, trichinosis, toxoplasmosis, Lyme disease, and leptospirosis), drug abuse (alcohol, heroin, cocaine, and methamphetamines), or as peripartum cardiomyopathy.

3.1. Pathophysiology

Dilated cardiomyopathy presents with a decrease in LV ejection fraction (LVEF) as described earlier, congestive heart failure (CHF) or as ventricular arrhythmias. Initially, the ventricle dilates to increase the force of contraction and stroke volume in order to maintain the cardiac output (Frank-Starling law); however, as the disease progresses, these compensatory mechanisms gradually fail, leading to the ventricular failure and ultimately failure to maintain the cardiac output (CO).

3.2. Signs and symptoms

The patients of dilated cardiomyopathy present with symptoms like dyspnea, orthopnea, fatigue, weakness, and oedema in the lower extremities. Physical findings are similar to those seen in CHF. Some patients complain of dyspnea on exertion that may look like angina pectoris. Patients may have jugular venous distention, crepitation on auscultation, resting tachycardia, audible s3 and s4 heart sounds, pulmonary oedema, and cardiomegaly. Mitral and/or tricuspid regurgitation may be audible clinically if the ventricular dilation is marked.

The ECG may show ST-T segment abnormalities, atrial fibrillation, intraventricular conduction defects, and PVCs. The echocardiography reveals dilated cardiac chambers, global hypokinesia, low EF/fractional shortening, raised LVEDP, mitral or tricuspid regurgitation and/or mural thrombi. Right-sided cardiac catheterisation using a Swan Ganz Catheter reveals a high pulmonary capillary wedge pressure, high systemic vascular resistance, and a low cardiac output. Additional laboratory tests carried out may reveal raised brain natriuretic peptide levels.

3.3. Treatment

Management of DCM begins with lifestyle modifications such as adequate rest, weight control, low sodium diet, fluid restriction, stopping alcohol intake and smoking, and less physical activity during periods of cardiac decompensation.

Medical management: The patients of DCM are at increased risk of pulmonary and systemic thromboembolisation due to stasis of blood in the dilated hypokinetic cardiac chambers. Anticoagulation therapy with warfarin or dabigatran is often indicated in these patients. The risk of embolisation is the highest in patients with atrial fibrillation, severe left ventricular dysfunction, a previous history of thromboembolism, or echocardiographic evidence of a mural thrombus. Other medications like angiotensin-converting enzyme inhibitors and angiotensin antagonists, diuretics, beta blockers, vasodilators, digoxin, antiarrhythmics, and statins can be prescribed to keep the condition under control.

Patients with a LVEF <30% and an intraventricular conduction defect with wide QRS complex ≥130 ms may lack synchronised contraction of both ventricles. Resynchronisation of right and left ventricle with biventricular pacing using a cardiac resynchronisation therapy device (CRT-D) can restore synchronous contraction of both ventricles, shorten the QRS interval, decrease left ventricular size and improve systolic function, stroke volume and the overall survival rate of patients.

Heart transplantation is the definitive treatment and the most common indication for transplantation in patients with DCM for both adults and children. Patients that are likely to benefit highly from a heart transplant include patients who were previously very active, <60 years of age who show intractable symptoms of congestive heart failure despite optimal medical therapy.

3.4. Prognosis

Symptomatic patients with DCM who are referred to tertiary medical centres for care have a high 5-year mortality rate (50%). If the cardiomyopathy involves both the right and left ventricles, the prognosis is very poor. Haemodynamic abnormalities that predict a poor prognosis include:

- an ejection fraction <25%,
- pulmonary capillary wedge pressure > 20 mm Hg,
- cardiac index <2.5 L/min/m^2,
- pulmonary hypertension,
- systemic hypotension, and
- an increased central venous pressure.

3.5. Anaesthetic management for non-cardiac surgery

Any major surgeries on these patients can be associated with morbidity and mortality, therefore, requires planning. Optimisation of congestive heart failure (CHF) at least for a week before the planned surgery is advisable. In critically ill or patients undergoing a high-risk procedure or those in which CHF is not appropriately managed, intra-arterial BP line should be inserted preoperatively. Premedication should be tailored according to the patient's requirement and may include short acting anxiolytic and/or sedative. Regional anaesthesia or nerve blocks alone or in combination with general anaesthesia can help us achieve the set goals of anaesthesia with a minimal haemodynamic compromise. However, the ongoing anticoagulation therapy may limit the option of regional anaesthesia. American Society of Regional Anaesthesia (ASRA) guidelines must be strictly followed if the patient is on an anticoagulation therapy.

The goals of anaesthesia are to [4]:

- minimise any negative inotropic effect of anaesthetic drugs.
- prevent increases in afterload.
- maintain preload despite increased left ventricular end-diastolic pressure.
- maintain perfusion and control arrhythmias,
- avoid hypotension and tachycardia.
- avoid overdose of medications during induction as the circulation time of drugs is slow.

These patients can become haemodynamically unstable due to the depressant effect of anaesthetic agents, fluid shifts and ongoing blood loss, which add to the already poor myocardial function due the cardiomyopathy. Propofol, thiopentone and inhalational agents cause vasodilation and myocardial depression. Benzodiazepines like midazolam and nitrous oxide may cause cardiovascular depression. Etomidate, ketamine, and narcotics like opioids are the ones that have minimal adverse haemodynamic response. We need to use a balanced anaesthetic technique. Slow induction should be carried out. Response of induction agents may be delayed due to prolonged circulation time, so slow and titrated doses of anaesthetic agents should be administered. Additional doses may not be required.

Optimal pain management helps to maintain haemodynamic stability. Regional anaesthesia may be a source of excellent postoperative pain relief, reducing the episodes of sympathetically mediated tachycardia, and afterload increases.

Monitoring: In addition to basic monitoring, central venous pressure (CVP) monitoring allows us to measure preload and central venous saturation (ScVO$_2$). It provides for an access to administer inotropes and vasoconstrictors if needed. Direct intra-arterial pressure monitoring enables early identification of haemodynamic alterations by beat-to-beat measurement of BP. Pulmonary artery pressure monitoring is useful in patients undergoing high-risk or emergency surgery or those in whom large fluid shifts are anticipated. The role of noninvasive methods to estimate cardiac output as well as estimate global end-diastolic volumes, the extravascular lung water, and other indices if available are invaluable for assessing cardiac function.

Transesophageal echocardiography (TEE) is also helpful as it identifies causes of hypotension, response to fluid therapy or inotrope support, estimates preload, cardiac output, diastolic dysfunction, valve function, and regional wall motion abnormalities.

4. Hypertrophic cardiomyopathy

Hypertrophic cardiomyopathy can be defined as abnormal LV thickening without chamber dilation that is usually asymmetrical, develops in the absence of an identifiable cause (e.g. aortic valvular stenosis[AS] and hypertension), and is associated with myocardial fibre disarray.

Hypertrophic cardiomyopathy (HCM) is very common and can affect people of any age group. It affects both sexes equally. It is a cause of sudden cardiac arrest and death in apparently healthy young people, including young athletes. HCM is a relatively common inherited disorder with an autosomal dominant pattern of inheritance with variable expression and has a prevalence of 1 in 500.

Defects of at least 11 genes and >1440 mutations sites demonstrate its genomic heterogeneity.

4.1. Pathophysiology

The underlying structural abnormalities in HCM are:

1. myocardial cell disarray where the cells are rearranged in a disorganised pattern as opposed to a normal parallel myocyte arrangement;

2. coronary microvasculature dysfunction due to increased wall to lumen ratio; and.

3. remodelling changes occurring in the heart.

These changes in HCM patients lead to diastolic dysfunction, impaired coronary reserve, supraventricular and ventricular dysrhythmias, and sudden cardiac arrest. Left ventricular remodelling can include fibrosis, focal, diffuse, asymmetric, or concentric hypertrophy, as well as decrease in the cavity size. The most common subtype of HCM presents as hypertrophy of the septum and the anterio-lateral free wall.

LV outflow tract obstruction (LVOTO) occurs in HCM, and initially it was proposed that the basal septal hypertrophy encroaching on the LVOT caused the obstruction of the tract. However, more recent studies have pointed towards the fact that during ventricular systole, flow against an abnormally positioned mitral valvular apparatus results in a Venturi effect on the anterior leaflet of the mitral valve and induces systolic anterior movement (SAM) of the anterior mitral valve leaflet. The mitral valve apparatus abnormalities can include hypertrophied papillary muscles touching the septum, elongated mitral leaflets, anterior displacement of papillary muscles, or anomalous insertion of the papillary muscle onto the anterior mitral leaflet. LVOTO can be precipitated or aggravated by increased contractility of the heart or tachycardia or decreased end-diastolic volume or systemic vascular (arterial) resistance. With HCM, incidence of diastolic dysfunction is more than LVOTO.

Myocardial ischaemia is present in patients with HCM, irrespective of the presence or absence of coronary artery disease. Myocardial ischaemia is precipitated by several factors including

- a mismatch between ventricular mass and coronary artery size,
- increased oxygen consumption due to hypertrophy,
- abnormal coronary arteries,
- decreased diastolic filling time,
- increased LVEDP compromising coronary perfusion, and
- the presence of a metabolic derangement regarding the utilisation of oxygen at the cellular level.

Supraventricular or ventricular dysrhythmias are relatively common in these patients due to the presence of disorganised cellular architecture, expanded interstitial matrix and myocardial scarring. They are the cause of incidence of sudden arrest in this group of cardiomyopathy.

4.2. Signs and symptoms

The clinical presentation of HCM varies widely. These patients can present early in their life with debilitating symptoms or can live for decades asymptomatically while some others die suddenly. The most frequent symptoms include dyspnea, dizziness, exercise intolerance, angina, syncope, and/or sudden death.

Physical examination may be normal at rest but may reveal a double apical impulse, gallop rhythm, a systolic murmur and thrill in the presence of functional LVOTO. It is rare, but some people with hypertrophic cardiomyopathy can suffer sudden cardiac arrest during a vigorous physical workout. The physical activity can trigger dangerous arrhythmias leading to sudden death.

The major risk factors for sudden cardiac death are:

- a family history of sudden death;
- unexplained syncope;
- extreme hypertrophy of the left ventricular wall (0.30 mm);
- non-sustained ventricular tachycardia (VT)

Electrocardiography (ECG) changes include left atrial (LA) enlargement, pathologic Q waves, high QRS voltage complexes, ST segment depression, and inverted T waves in at least two or more consecutive leads.

Echocardiography can easily demonstrate the presence of myocardial hypertrophy. Ejection fraction is usually >80%, reflecting the increase in force of contraction of the heart. Echocardiography can also assess the mitral valvular apparatus, the presence of mitral regurgitation, and the presence of LVOTO by demonstrating turbulent flow across the aortic valve. Pressure gradients across the LVOT can be measured. Echocardiography is useful in evaluating diastolic function of the heart.

Invasive measures like cardiac catheterisation allow direct measurement of the increased left ventricular end-diastolic pressure and the pressure gradient between the left ventricle and the aorta.

The definitive diagnosis of HCM can be made by an endomyocardial biopsy and DNA analysis, but these diagnostic modalities are usually reserved for patients in whom the diagnosis cannot be established by non-invasive means.

4.3. Treatment

The varied clinical profile of HCM makes it difficult to establish some precise guidelines for the treatment of this condition. The treatment plan should be titrated according to individual patient requirements. However, it is prudent to mention that the patients who are at high risk for sudden death should receive aggressive treatment.

Medical management: Pharmacotherapy is aimed at reducing LVOTO, improving diastolic filling, and possibly decreasing myocardial ischaemia. A variety of medical therapies have been used in these patients with the aim of altering the natural history. These include β-blockers, Ca^{2+} channel antagonists (verapamil or diltiazem), and disopyramide regimens, all of which seem to be effective as compared to no treatment in HCM patients. Most of these drugs used help HCM patients to improve their symptoms by reducing or eliminating the LVOT pressure gradient. These medications also reduce LVOTO during exercise by blunting the sympathetic response and are thus useful in treating the symptoms and attenuating the risk of sudden cardiac arrest. Atrial fibrillation often develops in these patients. It is associated with an increased risk of thromboembolism and congestive heart failure. Amiodarone is the most effective drug for prevention of repeated episodes of atrial fibrillation in these patients. Long-term anticoagulation is indicated in the patients with recurrent or chronic atrial fibrillation to prevent thromboembolic episode reducing the mortality and morbidity associated with it.

More recently, perhexiline, which augments myocyte energy supply, has been shown to improve diastolic dysfunction and symptomatology, but detailed studies are yet to follow.

Alcohol septal ablation [5]: Ethanol can be infused into the septal branches of the left anterior descending coronary artery and induce a targeted septal myocardial infarction (MI). Alcohol septal ablation is associated with some serious hazards, most common being the right bundle branch block, which has a post-procedural incidence of approximately 50%. Other complications include remote MI due to collateral circulation or an ethanol injection into the incorrect coronary, coronary dissection, ventricular septal rupture, heart failure, and heart block.

Surgical management: The American and European Colleges of Cardiology recommend myectomy in patients with:

1. labile obstruction and peak LVOT pressure gradients ≥50 mm Hg during exercise or provocation and resting gradients >30 mm Hg and.

2. NYHA class II through IV symptoms refractory to medical therapy.

Some patients may be candidates for implantable cardioverter-defibrillator (ICD) implantation while as principal surgical option is surgical myomectomy.

Prognosis: The overall mortality rate of HCM is 1% per annum. However, some patients at higher risk of sudden death as described before have an annual mortality rate of 5%.

Patients undergoing non-cardiac surgery: Most of the time, the patients with HCM are asymptomatic when they show up in the PAC clinic for elective surgeries. In the absence of signs and symptoms, the ECG findings may suggest that the patient has underlying HCM.

Initial patient evaluation should be aimed at determining the disease severity by assessing functional status of the patient, personal and family cardiac history, the presence or absence of cardiac and respiratory symptoms, history of rhythm disturbances, current medications, and previous strokes, or congestive heart failure history. During physical examination, all murmurs should be evaluated for dynamic changes with rest and exertion, and patients with murmurs that do not fulfil the criteria of a benign murmur should undergo an echocardiographic examination before surgery. Patients should be instructed to continue their rate controlling medications and maintain proper hydration preoperatively. Moreover, the presence of an automatic ICD and if it has been recently checked should be determined.

Preoperative management: A lot of patients with HCM may experience perioperative cardiac events like MI, congestive heart failure, severe hypotension, and supraventricular and ventricular tachydysrhythmias. Therefore, we need to focus on understanding the basic pathophysiology of the events and adjust our anaesthetic plans according to the patient needs.

In patients with HCM, preoperative administration of anti-anxiety medications may help to reduce anxiety and prevent the activation of anxiety-induced sympathetic response. Adequate preoperative intravenous fluid administration may help in preventing LVOTO and minimise the effect of positive pressure ventilation on central blood volume.

For patients who have an ICD in situ, the device should be turned off just before the surgery and an external defibrillator should be readily available and the ICD should be positively reactivated in the recovery room.

The anaesthetic goals are [4]:

- maintenance of sinus rhythm;
- reduction in sympathetic activity to reduce chronotropy and inotropy;
- the maintenance of systemic vascular resistance;
- maintenance of left ventricular filling.

Tachycardia, arrythmias, and decreases in afterload will exacerbate LVOTO and may cause haemodynamic deterioration. In addition to this, increases in contractility (chronotropy) and decreases in preload will accentuate LVOTO. Therefore, the principle of treatment for hypotension is volume expansion (including increasing preload in the Trendelenburg position) and use of drugs that increase systemic vascular resistance without a positive inotropic or chronotropic response (e.g. phenylephrine and vasopressin). Sympathetic response secondary to patient anxiety, intubation process, and surgical site incision and acute changes in preload, afterload, and contractility secondary to the pharmacological effects of anaesthetic agents, blood loss during surgery, and postoperative pain can precipitate haemodynamic collapse. DC cardioversion may be necessary in case of sudden onset of atrial fibrillation that is haemodynamically unstable.

Although both general and neuraxial anaesthesia can be used, it is important to have a clear understanding of the haemodynamic changes associated with each option. Depending on the route of the anaesthetic drugs chosen, close monitoring and titration of the medications affecting heart rate, preload, afterload, contractility of myocardium, and sympathetic activity are important. Neuraxial techniques may also be considered. In general, a slow controlled titration of medication via an epidural is preferred over a single dose spinal anaesthesia with the aim of maintaining preload and afterload and avoiding sympathetic stimulation. Regional anaesthesia can be an invaluable tool to manage postoperative pain and in turn prevent the activation of sympathetic response in these patients.

In addition to the standard American Society of Anaesthesiologists monitoring requirements, an intra-arterial catheter and/or non-invasive pulse plethysmographic variability (PPV) index monitor and central venous pressure (CVP) monitoring may be considered. The overall haemodynamic goals include maintaining the mean arterial blood pressure at >65–70 mm Hg to maintain coronary perfusion pressure to the subendocardium in the hypertrophied heart. The most useful monitoring tool for patients undergoing high-risk surgery is TEE. TEE can determine whether haemodynamic alterations are caused by hypovolemia, increased LVOTO or SAM, or LV systolic dysfunction.

Postoperative management: Patient with HCM should be continuously monitored in the postoperative room. All factors that activate a sympathetic response like pain, hypothermia, shivering, anxiety, hypoxia, and hypercarbia should be immediately addressed. The maintenance of euvolemia and prompt treatment of hypotension is very important.

5. Restrictive cardiomyopathy

Restrictive cardiomyopathy (RCM) is a disorder of the myocardium that occurs due to increased myocardial stiffness (decreased compliance) that leads to impaired ventricular filling. Size of both ventricle chambers and systolic function usually remains normal or near-normal until later stages of the disease. RCM may arise as a result of either inherited or acquired predispositions and diseases or a combination of the both, and can broadly be classified as infiltrative, non-infiltrative, storage disease, and endomyocardial fibrosis. Restrictive cardiomyopathy is prevalent in tropical regions of the world, where incidence of endomyo-cardial fibrosis is high. In non-tropical regions, idiopathic fibrosis is the common cause and is associated with increasing age. Other rare causes of RCM include amyloidosis, haemochromatosis, sarcoidosis, and eosinophilic endocarditis.

5.1. Pathophysiology

RCM is characterised by contracted stiff ventricles with progressive impairment of diastolic filling, leading to the haemodynamic problem of a low preload but high ventricular filling pressure. This pattern of diastolic dysfunction leads to dilation of the atria and elevation of mean atrial pressures, resulting in biventricular "backward heart failure" manifesting itself as pulmonary venous congestion leading to dyspnea as well as systemic venous pressure elevation resulting in peripheral oedema. Systolic function is preserved in most cases. However, in spite of intact systolic function, the restrictive pathology on true ventricular preload limit the stroke volume, resulting in low cardiac output and ultimately hypoperfusion of the tissues.

5.2. Signs and symptoms

RCM presents with signs and symptoms of both right and left heart failure. Patients complain of exercise intolerance because of diminished cardiac output. Patients often have a low volume pulse, an audible third heart sound, regurgitant murmurs, and a raised JVP with rapid X and Y descent that increases or fails to decrease on inspiration. Low blood pressures are often seen, complicating heart failure management. Pulmonary oedema is uncommon. Syncope occurs occasionally, often exertional, reflecting the limited ability of the heart to increase diastolic filling and is an ominous sign. Syncope may also be aggravated by antihypertensive medications. Concomitant autonomic neuropathy can precipitate orthostatic hypotension as can volume contraction from nephrotic syndrome.

Arrhythmias and conduction disturbances are frequent. Less frequent cardiac manifestations include dynamic LV outflow obstruction, often confused with hypertrophic cardiomyopathy; cardiac ischaemia caused by amyloid deposition in intramural coronary arteries; and intracardiac thrombosis caused by atrial wall standstill, with a risk for systemic embolisation.

The ECG may demonstrate conduction abnormalities. The chest X-ray shows signs of pulmonary congestion and/or pleural effusion, but cardiomegaly is absent. Echocardiography-based two-dimensional and Doppler are essential for determining diastolic dysfunction and for distinguishing patients with RCM from patients with restrictive physiology because of constrictive pericarditis. Echocardiography may also provide information to suggest a specific diagnosis such as the presence of regional wall motion abnormalities in a non-coronary distribution and aneurysms, which would raise the suspicion for cardiac sarcoidosis (CS). Cardiac magnetic resonance (CMR) imaging can aid in the diagnostic process, but the use should be determined on an individual basis. Endomyocardial biopsy (EMB) may be helpful for establishing a diagnosis in some cases. Ultimately, diagnosis of any of the RCMs relies on a constellation of clinical, laboratory, and imaging findings.

5.3. Management

Medical management: Treatment of RCM includes treating the underlying cause (if identified) and heart failure management. Diuretics are the mainstay of treatment to reduce volume overload. However, volume status in patients with RCM may be challenging to manage, as patients with RCM rely on high filling pressures to maintain cardiac output and excessive diuresis may result in tissue hypoperfusion. Digoxin must be used with great caution because it is potentially dysrhythmogenic in patients with amyloidosis. The use of β-blockers or calcium channel blockers to increase filling time or to manage arrhythmias should be carefully introduced, as some patients may be intolerant. Angiotensin-converting enzyme inhibitors and angiotensin II receptor blockers may also be considered, but the proof of benefit is lacking, and these agents may not be well tolerated. Anticoagulation is required in patients with atrial fibrillation, mural thrombus, or evidence for systemic embolisation and may be helpful in most patients because of propensity for thrombus formation in the left atrial appendage.

Surgical management: No corrective surgery has yet been proposed that would be 100% effective in improving the heart function in RCM. Advanced heart failure therapies, including cardiac transplantation, may be beneficial for selected patients. Heart transplantation is the only effective surgery that can be offered to the patients with restrictive cardiomyopathy. It may be the best option for those who are already symptomatic at the time of diagnosis or in whom reactive pulmonary hypertension exists. Left ventricular assist device (LVAD) therapy may be particularly applicable in patients with RCM as a bridge to transplant or as definitive therapy.

5.4. Patients posted for non-cardiac surgery

RCM presents a huge challenge for anaesthetists due to the high risk of morbidity and mortality. General anaesthesia causes vasodilation, suppresses the myocardium, and reduces venous return. The latter can be worsened by intermittent positive pressure ventilation resulting in cardiac arrest. Invasive arterial blood pressure monitoring and transesophageal echocardiography are useful in identifying the causes of cardiovascular instability [6].

The overall aims of anaesthesia are:

- sinus rhythm to be maintained if possible;
- to maintain adequate filling pressures;
- to maintain SVR in the presence of relatively fixed cardiac output.
- to manage electrolyte disturbances;
- to use anaesthetic agents with minimal cardiovascular effect like ketamine or etomidate.

6. Arrhythmogenic right ventricle cardiomyopathy

Arrhythmogenic right ventricle cardiomyopathy (ARVC) is characterised by structural abnormalities and cardiac dysfunction of mainly the right ventricle, but it can also involve the left ventricle. It is a rare type of cardiomyopathy. It occurs if the muscle tissue in the right ventricle dies and is replaced by a scar tissue. This disrupts the pathway of the heart's electrical signals leading to arrhythmias.

ARVC usually affects teenagers or young adults. ARVC has a prevalence of 1 in 5000 among healthy young people. ARVC is seen in up to 20% of all causes of sudden death in young people. It is a complex genetic condition due to its genetic variation.

6.1. Pathophysiology

Histologically, the myocardial cells are replaced by the adipose and fibrous tissues. These alterations can form a re-entry electrical circuit triggering arrhythmias. ARVC usually starts as a localised disease with regional wall abnormalities. As the disease progresses, the right ventricle continues to lose the healthy tissue and dilates and becomes thin walled. Patients can develop right bundle branch block before they finally present with the symptoms of right ventricular failure between the fourth and fifth decades of life.

6.2. Signs and symptoms

Young patients often present with syncope, arrhythmia, cardiac arrest, or sudden death. The diagnosis of ARVC should be considered in:

- Young male athletes with cardiac symptoms.
- ECG showing ventricular tachycardia with left bundle branch block morphology.
- T-wave inversion in leads V1–V3.
- Premature ventricular complexes with left bundle branch block morphology.
- Spontaneous non-sustained ventricular tachycardia.

An accurate diagnosis of ARVC is important due to the high risk of drug-resistant arrhythmias and sudden cardiac death. The diagnosis can be established by myocardial biopsy, which shows adipocytes and fibrous tissue. However, these changes can be localised and may not be present at the exact site of biopsy. The availability of cardiac MRI and the gadolinium enhancement techniques are now fundamental in diagnosing ARVC eliminating the need for biopsies.

6.3. Management

The main aim of medical management is to prevent or reduce the risk of fatal arrhythmias.

- Sotalol, verapamil, and amiodarone can be used.
- Due to the recurrence of arrhythmias and drug resistance, continuous Holter monitoring, or an electrophysiological study may be required. Catheter ablation can be used as a palliative rather than a curative intervention. It is indicated in patients with monomorphic VT due to alocalised ARVC, with a drug-resistant arrhythmia, or with frequent intervention following ICD implantation [7].

- Early placement of an ICD may be lifesaving.

- In some exceptional cases, heart transplantation may be required.

7. Peripartum cardiomyopathy

Peripartum cardiomyopathy is a rare, dilated form of cardiomyopathy of unknown cause that occurs during the peripartum period, that is, the third trimester of pregnancy until 5 months after delivery. Peripartum cardiomyopathy (PPCM) is a major concern for anaesthetists and can occur in 1 in 10,000 pregnancies, but it is higher in subsequent pregnancies [8]. Patients may present with severe heart failure during the third trimester or up to 5 months postpartum. Many of these patients deliver via a normal vaginal delivery without complications; however, a few may require a Caesarean section.

Risk factors include maternal age > 30 years, multiparty, African descent, obesity, multiple pregnancy, hypertensive disorders, tocolytic therapy, viral infection, and cocaine use.

Diagnostic criteria of peripartum cardiomyopathy: The diagnosis of PPCM is usually made after the other causes of acute heart failure have been excluded. The criteria are:

- Heart failure developing towards the end of pregnancy or up to 5 months' postpartum

- Absence of another identifiable cause of cardiac failure

- Absence of cardiac symptoms or disease before late pregnancy

- Left ventricular dysfunction - defined as an EF <45% or reduced fractional shortening of <30%

7.1. Signs and symptoms

The patients usually present with sign and symptoms of heart failure: dyspnea, fatigue, and peripheral oedema. In early stages, these signs may mimic the presenting features of normal late pregnancy.

Echocardiography may show new onset of unexplained LV dysfunction and documentation of a new finding of dilated cardiac chambers with LV systolic dysfunction during the period surrounding parturition.

7.2. Treatment

The main aim of treatment is to relieve the symptoms of heart failure. Diuretics, vasodilators, and digoxin can be used effectively. During pregnancy, vasodilation is accomplished with hydralazine and nitrates. Intravenous immunoglobulin may have a beneficial effect. Thromboembolic complications are not uncommon, and anticoagulation may be required in most patients. Heart transplantation may be considered in patients who do not improve over time.

7.3. Prognosis

The mortality in this group of patients is as high as 30–60% due to pulmonary oedema and systemic embolisation with most deaths occurring mostly within 3 months of delivery.

7.4. Anaesthetic management

We have a very little literature regarding the anaesthetic management of PPCM yet. Optimum fluid management and avoiding myocardial depression are the major concerns for anaesthetists.

According to a few case reports, both general anaesthesia and neuraxial blocks have been successfully used for elective or emergency Caesarean section. Combined spinal epidural anaesthesia (CSE) is preferred by some. CSE causes less haemodynamic instability, has a higher success rate than epidural anaesthesia, results in better patient satisfaction, and provides good postoperative analgesia.

8. Takotsubo cardiomyopathy

Recently, Takotsubo cardiomyopathy has been described. Takotsubo cardiomyopathy is a rare condition of transient, reversible severe LV dysfunction and characterised by chest pain, dyspnoea, ST-T changes in ECG, ventricular arrhythmias, regional wall motion abnormalities on echocardiography, elevated cardiac enzymes, haemodynamic instability, pulmonary oedema, cardiogenic shock, or cardiac arrest without angiographic evidence of CAD.

8.1. Sign and symptoms

It is rare, usually occurs in postmenopausal women associated with stress and chest pain. ECG changes may include prolonged QTc interval which resolve in 1–2 days, ST-T changes, Q waves, resolve by discharge from hospital, and T inversion resolves slowly.

This condition is also known as apical ballooning syndrome and broken heart syndrome or stress-induced cardiomyopathy. Echocardiography shows akinesia of apical or midventricular segments leading to systolic dysfunction. The normal basal segments become hypercontractile, giving a ballooned-out appearance of the apical or mid-cavity segments. Ballooning may lead to altered spatial relationships between mitral leaflets and subvalvular apparatus, which may result in MR and dynamic LVOTO causing SAM.

Reversible myocardial ischaemia is seen on myocardial perfusion imaging, and positron emission tomography and magnetic resonance imaging confirm LV dysfunction. Biopsy may show lymphocytic infiltrates. Plasma levels of brain natriuretic peptide, catecholamines, cardiac enzymes and metanephrine are found to be elevated.

8.2. Management

Optimal therapy is yet to be defined [9]. Beta blockers, diuretics, and ACE inhibitor and vaso-dilators have been used. Adrenergic agonists and antiadrenergic therapy (beta adrenergic blockers or alpha 2 agonists) and QT prolonging medications are to be avoided.

8.3. Anaesthetic management

A principle anaesthetic goal is to avoid psychological and physical stress that could trigger acute cardiomyopathy in susceptible patients. Thorough patient counselling, effective premedication and preoperative beta blocker therapy before transfer to operating room are highly effective.

Laryngoscopy, intubation, extubation, emergence, and inadequate postoperative pain control may cause a sympathetic response and increase catecholamine levels, so an optimal anaesthesia/analgesia is required in these phases. It is suggested that regional anaesthesia may be beneficial, but adequate studies to support this theory are not available.

It is unclear whether administration of inotropic drugs to treat systolic dysfunction is harmful. Inotrope of choice remains unclear, though Milrinone, aphosphodiesterase inhibitor, and a calcium sensitizer, levosimendan are suggested. Mechanical support of circulation with IABP or LVAD is an option to tide over periods of crisis. Beta blocker therapy may not be haemodynamically tolerated or could be potentially hazardous. Beta agonists should be avoided or used carefully, vasopressors may be used and supportive treatment for CHF should be instituted. LV dysfunction resolves within 2–4 weeks. Most cases recover spontaneously with a mortality risk of 0–8%.Recurrence occurs in 2–5% cases [10].

9. Intensive care unit management

When a person is admitted with a diagnosis of cardiomyopathy, the main aims of therapy whether in the intensive care or coronary care unit are, to reduce the workload of the heart and to improve the pumping ability of the heart. This can be achieved with the help of drugs such as inotropes, diuretics, ACE inhibitors, beta blockers, calcium channel blockers, and so on, which aids in improving the pumping action of the heart muscle and treatment to ensure the proper volume of blood in the body.

Treatment of the patients in the intensive care unit depends not only on the type and the severity of cardiomyopathy but also condition of patient. Treatment may include conservative management with drugs, implantation of pacemakers, defibrillators for those prone to fatal heart rhythms, ventricular assist devices or extracorporeal membrane oxygenators for severe heart failure, or ablation for recurring dysrhythmias that cannot be managed by drugs or cardioversion. The goal of management in the intensive care unit is often symptomatic, and some patients may eventually require a heart transplant.

10. Conclusion

Nowadays, cardiomyopathies are being identified increasingly as a result of improved means of detection with echocardiographic examination and an increase in the ageing population group. In addition, the presentation of this disease is varied. It may be sudden or already well known to the patient. Anaesthesia administration for patients with cardiomyopathy can lead to perioperative morbidity and mortality during elective or, more importantly in emergency surgeries. Therefore, anaesthesia and postoperative care have to be carefully titrated, planned, and monitored for every patient, for which we need a thorough understanding of the patho-physiology of cardiomyopathies. The best approach would be a multidisciplinary team that includes anaesthetists, cardiologists, and surgeons. As anaesthesiologists, we have to expand our horizon from operating room to ICU with a thorough understanding of non-invasive and invasive monitoring methods and a basic knowledge of transthoracic echocardiography.

Abbreviations

AHA	American Heart Association
ARSA	American Society of Regional Anaesthesia
ARVC	arrhythmogenic right ventricular cardiomyopathy
AS	aortic stenosis
CAD	coronary artery disease
CHF	congestive heart failure
CMR	cardiac magnetic resonance
CO	cardiac output
CTR-D	cardiac resynchronisation therapy device
CVP	central venous pressure
DCM	dilated cardiomyopathy
EF	ejection fraction
EMB	endomyocardial biopsy
HCM	hypertrophic cardiomyopathy
IABP	intra-arterial blood pressure
ICD	implantable cardioverter-defibrillator

LA	left atrium
LV	left ventricle
LVAD	left ventricular assist device.
LVEDP	left ventricular end-diastolic pressure
LVEF	left ventricular ejection fraction
LVOTO	left ventricular outflow tract obstruction
NYHA	New York Heart Association
PPCM	peripartum cardiomyopathy
PPV	pulse plethysmographic variability
PVC	premature ventricular complex
RCM	restrictive cardiomyopathy
SAM	systolic anterior moment
$ScVO_2$	central venous oxygen saturation
SVR	systemic vascular resistance
TEE	trans esophageal echocardiography
VT	ventricular tachycardia
WHO	World Health Organisation

Author details

Nandita Mehta* and Sayyidah Aasima tu Nisa Qazi

*Address all correspondence to: drnanditamehta@gmail.com

Department of Anaesthesia and Critical Care, Acharya Shri Chander College of Medical Sciences and Hospital, Jammu, India

References

[1] Maron BJ, Towbin JA, Thiene G, Antzelevitch C, Corrado D, Arnett D, et al. Contemporary definitions and classification of the cardiomyopathies: An American Heart Association Scientific Statement from the Council on Clinical Cardiology, Heart Failure and Transplantation Committee; Quality of Care and Outcomes Research and Functional Genomics and Translational Biology Interdisciplinary Working Groups; and Council on Epidemiology and Prevention. Circulation. 2006;**113**:1807-1816

[2] Elliott P, Andersson B, Arbustini E, Bilinska Z, Cecchi F, Charron P, et al. Classification of the cardiomyopathies: A position statement from the European Society of Cardiology Working Group on myocardial and pericardial diseases. European Heart Journal. 2008;**29**:270-276

[3] Arbustini E, Narula N, Dec GW, Reddy KS, Greenberg B, Kushwaha S, et al. The MOGE(S) classification for aphenotype-genotype nomenclature of cardiomyopathy: Endorsed by the World Heart Federation. Journal of the American College of Cardiology. 2013;**62**:2046-2072

[4] Stoelting RK, Dierdorf SF. Cardiomyopathy. In: Stoelting RK, editor. Anaesthesia and Coexisting Disease. 3rd ed. New York: Churchill Livingstone; 1993. pp. 97-102

[5] Abozguia K, Elliott P, McKenna W, Phan TT, Nallur-Shivu G, Ahmed I, Maher AR, Kaur K, Taylor J, Henning A, Ashrafian H, Watkins H, Frenneaux M. Metabolic modulator perhexiline corrects energy deficiency and improves exercise capacity in symptomatic hypertrophic cardiomyopathy. Circulation. 2010;**122**:1562-1569

[6] Ammash NM, Seward JB, Bailey KR, et al. Clinical profile and outcome of idiopathic restrictive cardiomyopathy. Circulation. 2000;**101**:2490-2496

[7] Basso C, Corrado D, Bauce B, et al. Arrhythmogenic right ventricle cardiomyopathy. Circulation. Arrhythmia and Electrophysiology. 2012;**5**:1233-1246

[8] Shnaider R, Ezri T, Szmuk P, et al. Combined spinalepidural anesthesia for cesarean section in a patient with peripartum dilated cardiomyopathy. Canadian Journal of Anesthesia. 2001;**48**:681-683

[9] Banerjee S. Takotsubo cardiomyopathy: A review. JSM Atherosclerosis. 2016;**1**:1011

[10] Littlejohn FC, Syed O, Ornstein E, Connolly ES, Heyer EJ. Takotsubo cardiomyopathy associated with anesthesia: Three case reports. Cases Journal. 2008;**1**:227

4

Severe Acute Pancreatitis and its Management

Arshad Chanda

Abstract

Severe acute pancreatitis (SAP) is a severe form of acute pancreatitis, which requires often intensive care therapy. The common aetiology varies with geographic locations. In Middle East, biliary pancreatitis is the commonest type. Initial phase of the disease is due to profound release of the proinflammatory marker, then the organ dysfunction takes over. It mainly divided into three types depending upon the pathological changes that are oedematous, necrotic and haemorrhagic. The common clinical presentation is typical abdominal pain radiating to the back and relieved by typical positioning i.e. sitting or leaning forwards. Raised pancreatic amylase and lipase with imaging will help to diagnose the SAP. The outcome of SAP is dictated by various criteria and scores. The commonly used scoring systems are Ranson's and Glasgow scores, whereas the local complication is diagnosed and predicted by the Balthazar's score. The management of SAP is mainly analgesia, prevention of complications and supportive care. Initially, laparotomy was recommended routinely for SAP complicated by necrosis of the pancreas and continuous lavage, but nowadays, minimal invasive image guided drainage is the recommended modality. The most common complications of concern are the abdominal compartment syndrome, Acute respiratory distress syndrome (ARDS), and infection of the pancreatitis necrosis. SAP has a high mortality rate (up to 40%), but initial aggressive supportive management will improve the outcome.

Keywords: analgesia, Balthazar score, Glasgow score, image guided drainage, Ransom Score, severe acute pancreatitis

1. Introduction

Acute pancreatitis is an inflammatory condition of the pancreas with a wide spectrum of pathological and clinical manifestations. It ranges from mild and self-limiting condition to severe pancreatitis with multiorgan failure with high mortality [1, 2].

It was one of the most frequent gastrointestinal causes of hospital admissions in the United States with a total of 275,000 admissions in 2009. In the United Kingdom, hospitals serving a population of 300,000–400,000 people admit about 100 cases each year. Patients with severe acute pancreatitis need ICU admission and multidisciplinary team approach for treatment. It increases the health care cost enormously, and those survive will live with pancreatic endocrine and exocrine dysfunction.

This chapter will focus mainly on severe acute pancreatitis.

2. Definition

Acute pancreatitis is an acute inflammatory process of the pancreas. It is an acute condition presenting with abdominal pain and is usually associated with raised pancreatic enzyme levels in the blood or urine as a result of pancreatic inflammation. It is a disorder of the exocrine pancreas and is associated with acinar cell injury with local and systemic inflammatory responses [3].

3. Classification

There is a wide range of classifications for acute pancreatitis. The Revised Atlanta Classification in 2012 classified acute pancreatitis according to the severity of the disease, morphology and temporal relation [1, 3].

3.1. Classification according to the severity of pancreatitis

Acute pancreatitis is classified into three forms based on the severity [3].

1. Mild acute pancreatitis, which is characterized by the absence of organ failure and local or systemic complications.

2. Moderately severe acute pancreatitis, which is characterized by transient organ failure (resolves within 48 hours and without persistent organ failure >48 hours) and/or local or systemic complications.

3. Severe acute pancreatitis, which is characterized by persistent organ failure that may involve one or multiple organs.

3.2. Classification according to the phases of pancreatitis

Temporally, two phases of acute pancreatitis are as follows:

(i) Early-first week

Only clinical parameters are important for treatment planning and are determined by the systemic inflammatory response syndrome (SIRS), which can lead to organ failure.

(ii) Late-after the first week

Morphologic criteria based on CT findings combined with clinical parameters determine the care of the patient [4].

3.3. Classification according to the morphology of pancreatitis:

Morphologically, there are three types of acute pancreatitis as follows:

  (i) Acute oedematous (interstitial) pancreatitis

  (ii) Acute necrotizing pancreatitis

(iii) Haemorrhagic

Usually, the necrosis involves both the pancreas and the peripancreatic tissues, less commonly the peripancreatic tissues alone and rarely the pancreatic parenchyma alone [1].

The commonest cause in the western world is gallstones (50%) and alcohol (25%). Rare causes (<5%) include drugs (for example, valproate, steroids, and azathioprine), endoscopic retrograde cholangiopancreatography, hypertriglyceridaemia or lipoprotein lipase deficiency, hypercalcaemia, pancreas divisum and some viral infections (mumps and coxsackie B4). About 10% of patients have idiopathic pancreatitis, where no cause is found [5]. The aetiological factors are enumerated in **Table 1**.

Aetiology of Acute Pancreatitis	
Toxic Alcohol	Methyl alcohol Smoking Organophosphates Scorpion bite, certain spiders, Gila monster lizard
Mechanical obstruction/duct damage	Biliary pancreatitis—Cholelithiasis, Biliary sludge Malignancy—pancreatic, ampullary, cholangiocarcinoma Parasitic infections—ascariasis Periampullary diverticulum Penetrating duodenal ulcer, Duodenal obstruction
Trauma	Abdominal trauma—duct disruption
Metabolic	Hyperparathyroidism Hypertriglyceridemia Hypercalcaemia Diabetic ketoacidosis End-stage renal failure Pregnancy Post-renal transplant
Vascular	Necrotising vasculitis—SLE, Thrombotic thrombocytopenia Atheroma Shock
Immune-related—Auto-immune pancreatitis	Vasculitis—SLE, polyarteritis nodosa

Drugs	Corticosteroids, furosemide, tetracyclines, thiazides, oestrogen, valproic acid, Metronidazole, pentamidine, nitrofurantoin, erythromycin, methyldopa, ranitidine 5-ASA/salicylates, azathioprine/6-MP, didanosine, pentamidine, L-asparaginase
Infections	
Viral: Mumps, varicella-zoster, coxsackie, HSV, HIV	
Bacterial: Mycoplasma, Leptospira, Legionella	
Parasitic: Toxoplasma, cryptosporidium	
Fungal: As pergillus	
Miscellaneous/Idiopathic	Post-ERCP pancreatitis Pancreas divisum in some patients Ischaemia, hereditary pancreatitis is a rare familial condition

Table 1. Aetiology of acute pancreatitis.

4. Pathophysiology

The exact pathogenesis of acute pancreatitis is unknown, and there is an ongoing research at the molecular level. There are many pathophysiological hypothesis put forward to explain the processes. These hypotheses are based on the aetiology and risk factors. The final result of the pathophysiological process is activation of proteolytic enzymes (intra-acinar activation of trypsinogen) leading to breakdown of the junctional barrier between acinar cells and leakage of pancreatic fluid and enzymes into the interstitial space causing autophagy and autodigestion of acinar cells [2, 3]. **Diagram 1** depicts the hypothetical aetiopathogenic process of acute pancreatitis.

Three different phases can be seen during the pathogenesis of acute pancreatitis. The first phase is the acinar cell damage and death. The second phase is local inflammation of the pancreas. The third and final phase is the SIRS. The first two phases take place in the pancreas itself, while in the third phase causes the distant organ damage and extrapancreatic symptoms.

Pancreatic ductal obstruction and hypersecretion have been mentioned as factors that contribute to the initiation of the inflammatory process. Different pathophysiological mechanisms have been proposed for ethanol-induced pancreatitis. Explanations like ethanol-induced direct toxicity to the acinar cell, sphincter of Oddi dysfunction, hypertriglyceridaemia, free oxygen radical formation, and protein deposition within the pancreatic duct, which favours retrograde flow of enzymatic. These processes lead to activation of inflammation and membrane destruction. Newer hypotheses include ischaemia/reperfusion injury and enzymatic co-localisation. Post-endoscopic retrograde cholangiopancreatography (ERCP) pancreatitis: 1–3% develops pancreatitis, probably due duct disruption and enzyme extravasation. Patients at the risk of developing post-ERCP pancreatitis have sphincter of Oddi dysfunction or a history of recurrent pancreatitis, those who undergo sphincterotomy or balloon dilatation of the sphincter.

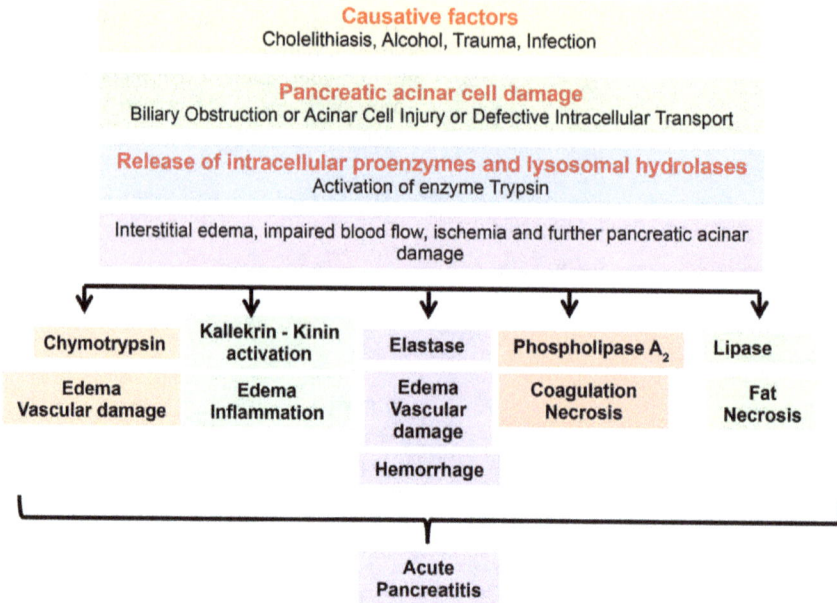

Diagram 1. Aetiopathogenesis of acute pancreatitis.

Systemic inflammatory response syndrome (SIRS) due to acute pancreatitis is because of the acinar cell death which releases activated pancreatic enzymes. This sets up a local inflammatory response which then activates systemic inflammatory response by release of cytokines, tumour necrosis factor, activation of immunocytes and the complement system activation [2–5].

5. Diagnosis of severe acute pancreatitis

5.1. Clinical presentation

Symptoms of acute pancreatitis are sudden onset of severe, persistent epigastric pain with or without radiation to the back. Radiation to the back is seen in about 50% of patients. It may be relieved by sitting or leaning forwards. Some patients complain of right upper quadrant pain. Pain is usually associated with nausea and vomiting.

5.2. Physical examination

Signs vary according to the severity of the disease. It ranges from mild epigastric tenderness to a diffusely tender abdomen.

Tachypnoea, tachycardia, and hypotension may be present. Fever due to inflammatory response. Acute swinging pyrexia suggests cholangitis. Icterus may be seen in biliary pancreatitis. Cullen sign, i.e. ecchymotic discoloration in the periumbilical area and Grey Turner sign, i.e. ecchymotic discoloration along the flanks due bleeding into the fascial planes, but these signs are not specific for acute pancreatitis. Abdominal distension due to ileus, guarding in the upper abdomen, free fluid may elicit shifting dullness. Pleural effusion is present in 10–20% of patients. Acute confusion due to metabolic derangement and hypoxaemia. Tetany is seen in some patient because hypocalcaemia [6, 7]

Perforated peptic ulcer, acute myocardial infarction, and cholecystitis should be rule out in differential diagnoses for acute pancreatitis.

5.3. Laboratory investigation

Serum amylase and lipase are both elevated in acute pancreatitis. The rise can be within 4–12 hours. The rise of >3 times the normal upper limit is the threshold for the diagnosis of acute pancreatitis [6, 7].

5.3.1. Serum amylase

It is an enzyme that hydrolyses the starch. The principal sources of amylase are the pancreas, salivary glands and fallopian tubes. Amylase has a shorter half life of 10 hours and returns to normal within 3–5 days. Hyperamylasaemia is seen in many other conditions. It may be increased in a number of other conditions like intestinal ischaemia and perforation, parotitis and acute renal failure, it is a less specific marker in acute pancreatitis. Its levels begin to rise 6–12 hours after the onset of acute pancreatitis, and they return to normal in 3–5 days. It has a high sensitivity (>90%) but a low specificity (as low as 70%) for the diagnosis of acute pancreatitis. Normal serum amylase level will not exclude acute pancreatitis if the patients present late to hospital [1, 6, 7].

5.3.2. Serum lipase

It a pancreatic enzyme that hydrolyses triglycerides. Its level increases within 4–8 hours of the onset and peaks at 24 hours and then returns to normal after 8–14 days. The rise in levels should be >3 times the upper limit of normal. It has excellent sensitivity in acute alcoholic pancreatitis. It is more specific than serum amylase for the diagnosis of acute pancreatitis. It has a sensitivity and specificity of 80–100% for acute pancreatitis. The principal sources of lipase are pancreas. The other sources are the tongue, liver, and intestine. These enzymes are useful in diagnosis of acute pancreatitis, but daily levels of these enzymes add no advantage in management. The levels are not useful in assessment of the severity of pancreatitis or decreasing levels are not marker of improvement. Simultaneous estimation of amylase and lipase levels does not improve accuracy [1, 6, 7].

5.3.3. Other lab data

In other laboratory investigations which help in etiological diagnosis are liver function test and serum triglycerides. Elevated liver enzymes, especially levels alanine transaminase Alanine Aminotransferase (ALT), level >150 U/L, it has a positive predictive value of 85% for gallstones. It will aid in diagnosis of acute biliary pancreatitis. Liver Function Test (LFT) should be done in all patients acute pancreatitis, patients within 24 hours of admission. C reactive Protein (CRP) levels will help in assessment of the severity of the disease process [5–7].

5.3.4. Imaging

The most commonly used imaging modalities in acute pancreatitis are transabdominal ultra-sound, endoscopic ultrasound, dynamic contrast enhanced CT scan and Magnetic Resonance Cholangiopancreatography (MRCP). Imaging studies are not indicated for diagnosing acute pancreatitis as it does not predict disease severity at the time of presentation to emergency department. Imaging studies are indicated when there is diagnostic dilemma due to non-con-clusive biochemical tests or because of the severity clinical condition or unexplained MODS, which warrants to rule out other intra-abdominal pathologies like gastrointestinal tract per-foration and peritonitis.

It also helps in rule out other conditions during the differential diagnosis of acute pancreatitis. The role of CT scan and magnetic resonance imaging (MRI) lies in the detection of complications of acute pancreatitis, such as pancreatic necrosis, peripancreatic fluid collections or pseudocysts; the presence of these complications can also be used to predict the severity of the disease [6].

5.3.5. Ultrasonography

5.3.5.1. Transabdominal ultrasound

Transabdominal ultrasound is less sensitive and less useful to visualize the inflamed or necrotic pancreas. The distended abdomen because of the gas-filled bowel obscures the pancreatic view. It cannot assess the extent of necrosis.

It helps in detection of gall stones, which are found in about 50% patients with acute pancre-atitis or dilatation of biliary tract secondary to obstruction.

Only indication of US scanning abdomen on presentation to emergency department is to rule out cholelithiasis as a cause for pancreatitis. Transabdominal ultrasound in later stages can help diagnosis of infection and therapeutic intervention-like guiding aspiration [6, 7].

5.3.5.2. Endoscopic ultrasonography

It is a combination of ultrasonography and endoscopic simultaneously. It is comparatively less invasive than endoscopic retrograde cholangiopancreatography (ERCP). It has a high sensitivity when compared to transabdominal ultrasound, especially in detecting the common bile duct microlithiasis and biliary sludge. It has a diagnostic yield of up to 88%. It helps in identifying patients who might benefit from endoscopic retrograde cholangiopancreatog-raphy and its therapeutic interventions. The added advantage of endoscopic ultrasonography is that it can be performed beside in unstable ICU patients, pregnant women where CT is contraindicated, and patients with metallic implants where MRCP is contraindicated [6, 7].

5.3.5.3. CT scan

Contrast-enhanced computed tomography is the gold standard to detect necrosis and to grade the severity of acute pancreatitis. This imaging modality also helps detecting local complication. CT scan findings range from localized oedema, pancreatic tissue inflammation (**Figure 1**), necrosis to extensive peripancreatic fluid collections (**Figure 2**).

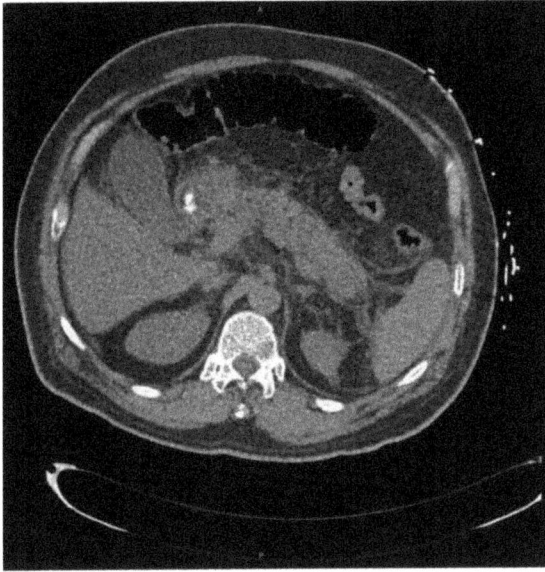

Figure 1. Oedematous pancreatitis.

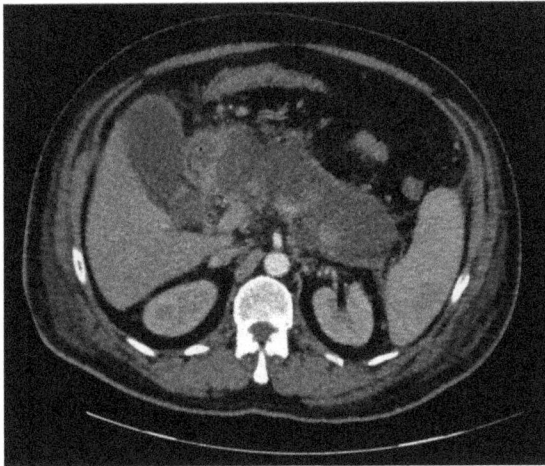

Figure 2. Pancreatitic necrosis.

CT findings of acute pancreatitis are diffuse or segmental enlargement of the pancreas due to interstitial oedema and irregular contour. Contrast non-enhancement represents pancreatic necrosis which is heterogeneous in appearance, peripancreatic fluid collection. Whole pancreatic necrosis is rare, multifocal areas are common. Necrosis is seen seen after 96 hours from the start of symptoms. CT scan performed before 72 hours will underestimate the degree of necrosis. The necrosis pancreas is variable involving the periphery with preservation of the core or involving the head, body, or tail separately or in combination. The outcome depends on the part of the pancreas involved. Necrosis of the entire pancreas has a relatively better outcome when compared to the head of pancreas involvement. Necrosis of the head of pancreas causes obstruction of the pancreatic duct there by an increase in pancreatic duct pressure causing to damage to acinar cells and leakage of destructive enzymes. Necrosis only in the distal portion of the pancreas has a favourable outcome and fewer complications [8]. **Figure 2** shows the CT image of pancreatic necrosis.

5.3.5.4. Efficacious use of computed tomography scanning in suspected acute pancreatitis

   (i) Patients in whom the clinical diagnosis is in doubt

  (ii) Patients with hyperamylasaemia and severe clinical pancreatitis **Figure 3** abdominal distension, tenderness, high fever (>39°C), and leucocytosis

 (iii) Patients with Ranson's score >3 or the acute physiology and chronic health evaluation (APACHE) II >8

  (iv) Patients showing lack of improvement after 72 hours of initial therapy,

   (v) Acute deterioration following the initial clinical improvement [8].

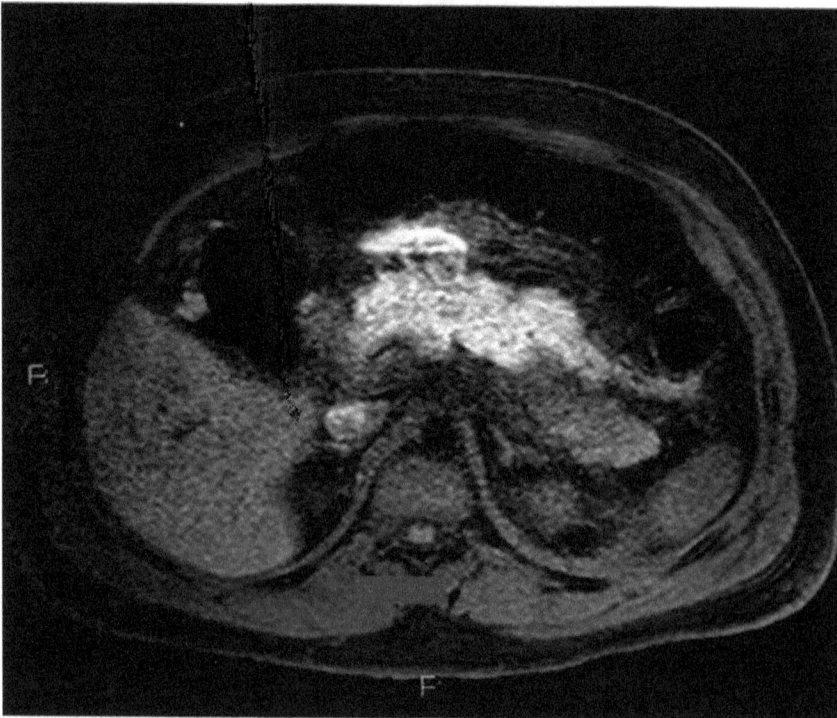

Figure 3. Haemorrhagic pancreatitis.

5.3.5.5. CT severity index

The modified CT severity index is a modification of the original CT severity index developed by Balthazar and colleagues in 1994. **Table 2** enumerates the details of the evaluation of Balthazar's computed tomography scoring system for acute pancreatitis.

The two factors that are useful in grading the severity of pancreatitis by CT are the extent pancreatic necrosis and the degree of peripancreatic inflammation. CT finding of necrosis and peripancreatic fluid collection strongly correlates with the complications (morbidity) and mortality [6, 7, 9, 10].

5.3.5.6. Grades of peripancreatic inflammation

(a) Normal pancreas

(b) Focal or diffuse pancreatic enlargement

(c) Pancreatic gland abnormalities associated with peripancreatic inflammation

(d) Single fluid collection

(e) Two or more fluid collections and/or gas present in or adjacent to the pancreas [10].

Inflammatory process	Grade	score
Normal	A	0
Focal or diffuse enlargement	B	1
Contour irregularity		
Inhomogeneous attenuation		
Grade B plus peripancreatic haziness/ Mottled densities	C	2
Grade B, C plus one ill-defined peripancreatic fluid collection	D	3
Grade B, C plus two ill-defined peripancreatic fluid collection or gas	E	4
Necrosis		
None	0	0
<30%	0	2
50%		4
>50%		6

Notes: Total score: Total points are given out of 10 to determine the grade of pancreatitis and aid treatment:
0–2: mild
4–6: moderate
8–10: severe.

Table 2. Evaluation of Balthzar's computed tomography scoring system for acute pancreatitis.

Repeat scanning is only indicated if there is any deterioration in clinical condition to rule out/ diagnose pancreatic necrosis, abscess or pseudocyst, haemorrhage, or bowel ischaemia or perforation.

5.3.5.7. Magnetic resonance imaging (MRI)

Magnetic resonance imaging (MRI) and MRCP are non-invasive imaging modalities. It has several advantages over CT, like no risk from radiation, can detect pancreatic duct continuity and parenchymal changes. It helps diagnose acute pancreatitis and identifying the aetiology of acute pancreatitis. MRI can accurately differentiate between necrotic and non-necrotic tissue.

5.3.5.8. Magnetic resonance cholangiopancreatography

It is especially useful to visualising the pancreatic duct and detecting lithiasis. MRCP is performed when ERCP has failed. The advantage of MRCP over CT scan is that iodinated contrast agents can be avoided and thereby avoid the risk for acute kidney injury.

Disadvantages of MRI and MRCP is transportation of critically ill patients to the MRI suite are limited access to patient during the acquisition of images and longer time to complete the study.

6. Assessment of severity

6.1. Why to assess the severity of the acute pancreatitis

1. To classify the disease process.

2. To predict the level of care needed, ICU or HDU for monitoring and supportive care.

3. To predict the outcome depending the severity of the acute pancreatitis, especially the mortality.

4. Select patients for specialised interventions as therapy to improve the outcome.

5. If patients are managed by the nonspecialist clinicians, then the scoring system will help them identify patients who need consultation and transfer to specialist centre.

6. For comparisons of severity within and between patient series.

7. In research for rational selection of patients for inclusion in trials.

8. It helps in intra-, inter-departmental and patient and patient family communication—using the same language.

Severity assessment should be carried out within 48 hours of diagnosis of acute pancreatitis. Patients with a body mass index over 30 are at higher risk of developing complications.

6.2. How to assess the severity of the acute pancreatitis

There are various scoring systems in vogue, using the clinical data, laboratory markers and radiological findings to assess and grade the severity of the acute pancreatitis. The scoring systems are of two types: one that correlates clinical features and lab indices and the other being the use of non-specific physiological scoring, namely, APACHE II and III. The commonly used scoring systems are the Ranson's criteria, Glasgow (Imrie) scoring systems, the APACHE II and III scoring systems (mainly used in ICU), the Simplified acute physiology score, bedside index of severity in acute pancreatitis (BISAP) scoring system, and the CT severity index. None of the scoring systems have a high sensitivity, specificity, positive predictive value or negative likelihood ratio. The scoring systems used at present are often inadequate in patients with severe Acute necrotizing pancreatitis (ANP), which is characterised by rapidly progressive multiple-system organ dysfunction [3, 4, 10].

6.3. Ranson's criteria

The Ranson's criteria were introduced in clinical practice in the early 1970s. It is the most widely used scoring system. Note that, 11 criteria are taken into account. **Table 3** enumerates the Ranson's criteria for assessment severity of acute pancreatitis. They were designed after analysis of 100 patients with alcohol-induced pancreatitis. It makes use of a combination of

---

Ranson's Criteria

Severity assessment

On admission

- Age > 55 years
- WBC > 16,000/μL
- Glucose > 11 (200 mg/dL)
- Lactate dehydrogenase (LDH) > 400 IU/dL
- AST > 250 IU/dL

After 48 hours

- Haematocrit fall > 10%
- Increase in urea > 1.8 mmol/L (>5 md/dL)
- Calcium < 2 mmol/L
- PaO_2 < 8 kPa (60 mmHg)
- Base deficit > 4 mmol/L
- Fluid deficit > 6 L

Risk factors mortality rate
0–2 < 1%
3–4 ≈ 15%
5–6 ≈ 40%
>6 ≈ 100%

Table 3. Ranson's criteria for assessment severity of acute pancreatitis.

clinical and biochemical parameters obtained at admission and during the first 48 hours after admission. It reflects the extent of metabolic derangement and estimates the risk for mortality.

Drawbacks of the scoring system are that the study was only for alcoholic pancreatitis, do not take into consideration the ongoing treatment and predicts high mortality which is not the case in today's practice.

The Ranson's criteria have a sensitivity 74%, specificity 77%, positive predictive value 49% and negative predictive value 91% [3, 4, 10].

6.4. Modified Glasgow criteria (Imrie score)

A decade after the Ranson's criteria were introduced, a re-evaluation of those criteria was done and found that the eight of the criteria were most predictive of the severity and outcome. **Table 4** enumerates the modified Glasgow criteria (Imrie score) for assessment severity of acute pancreatitis.

Those eight criteria were renamed as Glasgow criteria or Imrie score. It's use is limited in Emergency department (ED) as some of the variables are only evaluated at 48 hours. The criteria excluded from the Ranson's criteria are Lactate dehydrogenase (LDH), base deficit, and fluid deficit, and these were found to be least contributory in assessment of severity and outcome [9, 10].

The Glasgow (Imrie) criteria are valid for both alcohol induced and biliary pancreatitis. A scores 3 or more after 48 hours of presentation indicates severe acute pancreatitis.

6.5. Other markers of severity

6.5.1. C-reactive protein

It is an acute phase reactant. It should be done after 48 hours of presentation. It can be used both for the assessment of severity and monitoring the progress of the disease. Levels more than 100 mg/L late in the first week after presentation indicate that patient is developing pancreatic

---

Modified Glasgow criteria

On admission

- Age > 55 years
- WBC > 15,000/ μL
- Glucose > 10 ((no history of diabetes)
- PaO_2 < 8 kPa (60 mmHg)

After 48 hours

- Calcium < 2 mmol/L
- Serum albumin <32 g/L
- Lactate dehydrogenase (LDH) > 600 IU/dL
- AST/ALT > 600 IU/dL

Table 4. Modified Glasgow criteria (IMRIE SCORE) for assessment severity of acute pancreatitis.

necrosis. Procalcitonin will help identifying the pancreatic infection. IL-6, trypsinogen activation peptide, polymorphonuclear elastase, and carboxypeptidase B activation peptide can also be used for assessing the severity and monitoring the progress of the disease, but these are either used as a research tool or not yet routinely available.

Persistent high haematocrit is also an indicator of pancreatic necrosis and organ failure. If initial resuscitation is inadequate, then haemoconcentration is not a useful marker [3, 4, 10].

6.6. The acute physiology and chronic health evaluation (APACHE) II scoring system

The acute physiology and chronic health evaluation (APACHE) II is (Knaus et al.) used to quantify the severity of the illness in ICU patients. It contains 12 continuous variables, the age and the pre-morbid conditions (which reflect a diminished physiological reserve). Patients with an APACHE II score >8 have severe acute pancreatitis and are likely to develop organ failure. It can be used in monitoring the patient's response to therapy throughout the patient's hospital stay unlike Ranson's and Glasgow, which is assessed in the first 48 hours. Hence, it can assess both the severity and progress/deterioration. Disadvantages being that it is complex to perform and has been evaluated prospectively only in first 24–48 hours after the onset of pancreatitis. In criteria used, factors with most predictive value for mortality include advanced age, presence of renal or respiratory insufficiency and presence of shock. It has a sensitivity of 65%, specificity of 76%, positive predictive value of 43% and negative predictive value of 89%. APACHE III is also been used in predicting the severity of pancreatitis [10].

6.7. Bedside index of severity in acute pancreatitis (BISAP) score

BISAP score is a beside scoring system with fewer variables than Ranson's criteria. The data sued in scoring are the basic data recorded during the time of admission or taken from the first 24 hours of the patient's evaluation. **Table 5** enumerates the criteria of bedside index of severity in acute pancreatitis (BISAP) score for assessment severity of acute pancreatitis. It is a prognostic scoring system that predicts the mortality, whereas Ranson's score predicts

Bedside index of severity in acute pancreatitis (BISAP) score	Scores	
	1	0
BUN >25 mg/dL (8.9 mmol/L)	>25 mg%	<25 mg%
Abnormal mental status with a Glasgow coma score <15	Present	Absent
Evidence of SIRS (systemic inflammatory response syndrome)	2/4	Absent
Patient age	>60 years old	<60 years old
Imaging study reveals pleural effusion	Present	Absent

Table 5. Bedside index of severity in acute pancreatitis (BISAP) score for assessment severity of acute pancreatitis.

persistent organ failure. BISAP scores have the advantages over Ranson's and Glasgow scores of being calculated within 24 hours of admission, use fewer variables. BISAP score is higher in patients having SIRS, in older patients and in patients with altered mental status. It has the disadvantage that it cannot easily distinguish transient from persistent organ failure [3, 4, 10].

Patients with a score of zero predict a mortality of less than 1 whereas patients with a score of 5 predict a mortality rate of 22%. The way forward may be to use a combination of the Ranson's score, the radiological scoring systems and a descriptive organ failure score such as the sepsis-related organ failure assessment.

7. Management

Management of acute pancreatitis should be aggressive and begins early in the emergency department once the diagnosis is made. Initial resuscitation can affect the outcomes of acute pancreatitis significantly.

The treatment can be divided into three major parts as follows:

1. ICU admission and management

2. Treatment of the local complications

3. Treatment of the aetiology [2, 3, 8]

7.1. ICU/HDU admission

ICU/HDU admission is needed in patients with severe acute pancreatitis for close monitoring, organ support, and follow up. It is difficult to decide which patient is a candidate for ICU/HDU admission at the time of presentation. There is a lack of early and adequate predictors of impending organ dysfunction. But the patients present with signs of organ dysfunction like hypotension, respiratory insufficiency, coagulopathy (including Disseminated intravascular coagulation (DIC), and acute kidney injury are definite candidates for ICU/HDU admission. Other than organ dysfunction patients with severe metabolic derangements like hyperglycaemia, severe hypocalcaemia and patients with comorbidities like heart failure, chronic kidney disease where the acute on chronic organ dysfunction may develop are the candidates for ICU admission [10]

7.2. Monitoring

Monitoring a patient with acute severe pancreatitis can be divided into the following:

1. Monitoring of vital signs: Heart rate, blood pressure, respiratory rate, oxygen saturation, urinary output and level of consciousness

2. Biochemical evaluation of organ function: Blood gases, lactic acid, renal function test, coagulation profile, haematocrit, blood glucose and serum electrolyte levels, especially calcium,

magnesium, and liver function test. These test may alert impending organ dysfunction, improvement or worsening of the organ function

3. Development of local complications like pancreatic necrosis and infection, which are associated with increased morbidity and mortality.

    a. Pancreatic necrosis is detected by contrast enhanced CT scan

    b. Pancreatic infection needs repeated contrast enhanced CT scan with CT/US guided fine needle aspiration

4. Intra-abdominal pressure (IAP): Intra-abdominal hypertension (IAH) is related to the development of complications, especially necrosis and infection, bowel oedema. High IAP is one indication for intervention like aspiration or surgery [6, 7, 10].

7.3. Organ support

7.3.1. Cardiovascular dysfunction: hypotension and early fluid resuscitation

Hypotension is one of the most common presentations with acute pancreatitis. It is a sign of impending organ dysfunction. The hypotension is due to the third space loss secondary to the inflammatory response, this contributes to hypoperfusion and end organ perfusion dysfunction. Aggressive fluid resuscitation and rapid restoration of intravascular volume are the main stay of the treatment. It requires several liters of fluids. Both crystalloids and colloids can be used as resuscitation fluids. There is no evidence that colloids have any added benefit over crystalloids. Among the crystalloid, use of 0.9% sodium chloride is to be avoided. As it causes hyperchloraemic metabolic acidosis, which is associated with renal impairment, infections and activation of trypsinogen in a pH-dependent manner. Lactated Ringer's solution is a cystalloid, it is a balanced salt solution, It is fluid of choice it has been found to be less incidence of SIRS compared to normal saline. Both under resuscitation as well as over resuscitation can lead to adverse outcomes, hence very close monitoring is recommended. Over resuscitation can lead interstitial oedema, bowel oedema, Acute respiratory distress syndrome (ARDS) which can lead to organ dysfunction. Monitoring of fluids status should be done by physical examination (clinical condition, vital signs and urine output), volume responsiveness and dynamic parameters by sonography or invasive or semi invasive haemodynamic parameters. Metabolic indicators like serial measurements of blood urea nitrogen and haematocrit [11, 12].

7.3.2. Pulmonary dysfunction

Pleuropulmonary abnormalities are commonly associated with pancreatitis, respiratory dysfunction is rarely seen at the time of presentation to Emergency department (ED) but usually develops after fluid resuscitation. It manifests as acute lung injury or acute respiratory distress syndrome. It is one of the major components of multiple organ system dysfunction syndromes. Other manifestations are bilateral infiltrates, pleural effusion, pulmonary hypertension, and decreased thoracic compliance [11, 12].

7.3.2.1. Pulmonary management

Patients with acute severe pancreatitis should be monitored closely for early detection of failure. Respiratory support usually initiated by supplemental oxygen and mechanical ventilation is often required depending on the severity of respiratory dysfunction. Nasogastric decompression will decrease the distension and improve the compliance and prevent aspiration. Non-invasive ventilation is poorly tolerated in most of the patients because of abdominal distension and reduced functional residual capacity, careful selection of patient is warranted. Non-invasive ventilation is good choice to start with as it may avoid endotracheal intubation. Acute lung injury and Acute respiratory distress syndrome (ARDS) secondary to acute severe pancreatitis is similar to any other condition using lung protective strategies. Pleural effusion may need ultrasound-guided drainage. Good analgesia will help in chest physiotherapy, early physiotherapy will prevent atelectasis and related complications [11, 12].

7.3.3. Pain relief

Pain is one of the symptoms of acute severe pancreatitis. It causes discomfort and heightened sympathetic activity, impairment of oxygenation due to restriction of abdominal wall movement. Effective analgesia can be provided by the use of opioids and parenteral route, i.e. intravenous route is the preferred route. Analgesia may improve pulmonary dysfunction. In the past, morphine was supposed to exacerbate acute pancreatitis by promoting contraction of the sphincter of Oddi and increase pressure in the sphincter of Oddi dysfunction, but there is no good supportive evidence. Another modality of pain management is use of drugs like local anaesthetics through in epidural route [13, 14].

7.3.4. Nutrition support in acute pancreatitis

Acute pancreatitis is a catabolic and hypermetabolic pathophysiological condition. This disease process increases protein demand and the calorie requirements. This altered metabolic state is further deranged by poor oral intake due to pain, ileus or partial obstruction of the duodenum from pancreatic oedema. There are increased protein losses locally in the retroperitoneum due to inflammation and through pancreatic fistulae. These features may be compounded by the pre-existing malnutrition, e.g. in alcohol abuse [11, 12, 13].

If malnutrition and a prolonged negative nitrogen balance are not taken care, it may result in poor pancreatic healing, increased risk of infection, impaired immunity, gut dysfunction leading to translocation of bacteria. Nutritional care and therapy along with other therapeutics measures will results in faster recovery and better outcome.

Feeding during severe acute pancreatitis may be challenging. The questions to address during the initiation of the nutritional support are when? How? and what?

Earlier concept of feeding in acute pancreatitis: the pathogenesis of pancreatitis is assumed to be perpetuation of premature enzymatic activation. 'Resting the pancreas' the approach to avoid stimuli to exocrine secretion from the pancreas was thought to be most physiological method to treat the pancreatitis. Hence, parenteral nutritional was the preferred option to avoid stimulation of the inflamed pancreatic gland. The other hypothesis is that systemic inflammatory response syndrome is caused by the absorption of the pancreatic endotoxins and ultimately leads to multiorgan failure. If the gut mucosal barrier is maintained, then it reduces the absorption of endotoxin. The present concept of nutritional support in acute pancreatitis: the preferred route of nutritional support is 'enteral route', it should be initiated as early as possible within 24–48 hours of presentation. Parenteral route is second choice, especially if the presentation is severe and it is unlikely to start oral intake within the next 5–7 days. The advantages of the enteral feeding are improved gut blood flow, maintenance of mucosal integrity and barrier function there by reduction in microbial translocation and pancreatic infection, and better glycaemic control, avoidance of central venous access-related complications are benefits of enteral nutrition. There benefits are translated in lower incidence of infections, multiorgan failure and outcome, i.e. mortality and length of stay when compared to parenteral nutrition [11–13].

7.3.5. Route of enteral nutrition

If nutritional support is supplemented by the enteral route, then it is usually delivered by tube feeding. There is a controversy about nasogastric versus nasojejunal feeding. But there is not much evidence to support any one over the other. Though traditionally nasojejunal feedings (to be delivered distal to the ligament of Treitz) have been preferred with the concept of less stimulation of the exocrine pancreas, cholecystokinin (CCK) cells that are present in the distal third part of the duodenum get stimulated when food passing through duodenum. It releases CCK that stimulates the pancreas and increased volume of pancreatic enzymes and bicarbonate secretion. This may worsen the course of the disease. Nasogastric tube feedings have now been shown to as safe as the jejunal feeding. Nasogastric insertion can be at bedside. Fluoroscopy endoscopic (endoscopically placed guide wire) and specialist help is not needed. With the Nasogastric (NG) feeding, the standard precautions of aspiration like elevation of head end of bed should be followed.

The indication for nasojejunal feeds is when patients cannot tolerate gastric feeding due to ileus and slow bowel transit time. Nasojejunal (NJ) tube placement needs fluoroscopy, endoscopic, and specialist help. NJ tube may get displaced back into the stomach. Prokinetics and right-lateral positioning pass the tube through the into-duodenum. The correct positioning of the tube should be ascertained regularly by radiography [2, 7, 13].

7.3.6. Enteral nutritional supplements

No specific enteral nutrition supplement or immunonutrition formulation had any advantage. Low fat formulas with medium-chain triglycerides should be used enteral because it helps in better assimilation by direct absorption into the portal vein as there is lipase deficiency.

7.3.7. Complications of nutritional therapy

The common complications are metabolic and splanchnic. They are as follows:

Hyperglycaemia: Beta-cell death, peripheral insulin resistance irrespective of the route of feeding, needs monitoring of serum glucose and use IV insulin.

Hypertriglyceridemia is usually due to overfeeding. Monitor serum triglyceride level and titrate fat content.

Feed intolerance: Monitor abdominal pressure, bowel distension, residual volume and diarrhoea. Displacement of NJ tube [2, 9].

8. Pathogenesis of pancreatic infection and antibiotic prophylaxis

Infection is common in pancreatic necrosis, it occurs in approximately 40–70% of patients. Infection causes an increase in morbidity and mortality. There are various theories proposed for the mechanisms of infection in severe acute pancreatitis, namely bacterial translocation from the colon, via the biliary tree, especially in biliary pancreatitis, bacterial migration through the pancreatic duct from the lumen of the duodenum and haematogenous spread from bacteraemia due to other causes like infected central venous lines [5, 9, 10].

8.1. Role of antibiotic prophylaxis in severe acute pancreatitis

Prophylactic antibiotics in severe acute pancreatitis have been a topic of debate in the last 4–5 decades. Pancreatic necrosis more than 30% increases the chances of infection. The right choice of antibiotics is very important, those which have high penetration into pancreatic tissue. Carbapenems are both broad spectrum and excellent pancreatic penetration properties. Other antibiotics, which penetrate well in the pancreatic tissue, are cephalosporin, ureidopenicillins, fluoroquinolones, metronidazole and imipenem. Aminoglycosides have a poor penetration ability. Patients with mild pancreatitis do not benefit from antibiotics. In a meta-analysis by Sharma et al. [16], use of prophylactic antibiotics has shown mortality benefit in patients with Acute necrotizing pancreatitis (ANP) confirmed by contrast-enhanced CT (21–12.3%). Ref. [15, 16] prophylactic antibiotics use has not shown to decrease the need for interventional and surgical management but no effect on mortality.

8.2. Prophylactic antifungal therapy

Fungal infection in severe acute pancreatitis is associated with high morbidity and mortality.

It has been noted that the incidence depends on the severity of the disease, extent of necrosis and use of broad spectrum antibiotic administration. Prophylactic use of fluconazole has shown to be effective in decreasing the morbidity but not the mortality [10].

9. Treatment of local complications

9.1. Pancreatic necrosis and abscess

The presence of non-viable tissue in the pancreatic parenchyma, which is detected by the non-enhancement on the contrast-enhanced CT, is called as pancreatic necrosis. It can be focal or diffuse with associated peripancreatic involvement. It can be sterile necrosis or get infected in approximately 70% of the cases. The diagnosis of infection of the necrotic pancreas is diffi-cult. Infected necrosis is diagnosed in the patients who show no signs of improvement, signs of sepsis (leukocytosis and fever are confounded by the SIRS), worsening of clinical condi-tion, especially after improvement. The lab data to confirm the infection of the necrotic pan-creatic tissue are not reliable. Biomarker like CRP is usually high in severe acute pancreatitis, but procalcitonin can be used as a marker, but still it is not specific because in patients who are critically ill, there are other infection like Central Line-associated Bloodstream Infection (CLABSI), Ventilator-Associated Event (VAE) (Ventilator-Associated pneumonia (VAP)), Catheter-associated Urinary Tract Infections (CAUTI), etc. wherein procalcitonin is raised.

The best method to confirm the diagnosis of infected pancreatic necrosis is CT/US guided fine needle aspiration, Gram's staining, and culture. Multiple samples from all pockets should be taken or sampling needs to be repeated. Pancreatic abscess is a collection of pus in close proximity to pancreatic necrosis, which develops as a local infection of the necrotic pancreatic tissue after severe acute pancreatitis.

9.2. Management of sterile pancreatic necrosis

Sterile pancreatic necrosis is usually managed conservatively (non-operatively). Earlier in the 1990s, all necrotic pancreatitis use to undergo necrosectomy. Surgical intervention in sterile pancreatic necrosis may increase the risk of infection and thereby an increase in the mortal-ity. Patients with sterile pancreatic necrosis need close observation for evidence of infection. In selected patients with extensive necrosis may need surgical intervention if they do not improve for more than 6–8 weeks [3, 8, 11, 12].

9.3. Management of infected pancreatic necrosis pancreatic necrosis and abscess

Infected necrotic pancreatitis requires debridement and there is a consensus on surgical inter-vention in such cases. There is still a controversy about the best approach for debridement of the infected necrotic pancreatic tissue.

The aim of the intervention is removal of the infected necrotic substance. To achieve this goal, there are several techniques suggested. It ranges from drainage, debridement, lavage laparos-copy to laparotomy and packing.

9.4. Percutaneous drainage

- Anterior

- Retroperitoneal

This can be done when there are infected fluid collections or pus. It will be difficult to drain if it is just infected necrotic tissue or fluid/pus is too viscous. It has to be done CT/US guided and needs expertise. Complications are rare in expert hands. Usual complications with per-cutaneous drainage are bleeding, viscous perforation, fistula formation and super infection [3, 11, 12].

9.5. Surgical debridement/necrosectomy

- Minimally invasive

- Open surgical

These procedures can be performed transperitoneal or retroperitoneal which is decided on the location of necrosis and collections. Some patients need multiple sitting and planned relaparotomies. The open surgical approach carries higher risk of morbidity and mortality when compared to laparoscopic technique. There is higher risk of bleeding, perforation multiple organ failure, enterocutaneous fistula, incisional hernia, and new-onset diabetes mellitus [13, 14]

9.6. Management of the etiological factor

There is very few or nothing to do for the etiological management other than biliary pancreatitis. The treatments depend on the severity of the pancreatitis. In severe pancreatitis, there is no role of surgery. Surgery increases the morbidity and mortality. ERCP (endoscopic retrograde cholangiopancreatography) with sphincterotomy is indicated in patients with acute cholangitis. This will help in decreasing the pressure in pancreatic duct and lessens the severity of the disease. ERCP with sphincterotomy decreases the morbidity but not the mortality [13, 14].

10. Prevention of acute pancreatitis

Change in dietary habits and consumption of balance diet will prevent the gall stone formation, earlier cholecystectomy will prevent the recurrence of pancreatitis. Regular exercise, avoiding the high caloric intake, regular use of low fat diet will control the serum triglyceride levels and early introductions of statins will help in preventing the hyperlipidaemia associated pancreatitis. Moderation in alcohol intake will reduce the incidence of alcoholic pancreatitis [13, 14].

Author details

Arshad Chanda

Address all correspondence to: drarshadchanda@yahoo.com

Hamad General Hospital, Doha, State of Qatar

References

[1] Working Group IAP/APA Acute Pancreatitis Guidelines. IAP/APA evidence-based guidelines for the management of acute pancreatitis. Pancreatology. 2013;**13**:e1-e15

[2] Johnson CD, Besse MG, Carter R. Acute pancreatitis. British Medical Journal. 2014; **349**:4859. DOI: 10.1136/bmj.g4859

[3] Nirula R. Chapter 9: Diseases of the pancreas. In: High Yield Surgery. Philadelphia, PA: Lippincott Williams & Wilkins; 2000

[4] Clinical Practice and Economics Committee. AGA institute medical position statement on acute pancreatitis. Gastroenterology. 2007;**132**:2019-2021

[5] Ignatavicius P, Vitkauskiene A, Pundzius J, Dambrauskas Z, Barauskas G. Effects of prophylactic antibiotics in acute pancreatitis. HPB. 2012;**14**:396-402

[6] Wang GJ, Gao CF, Wei D, Wang C, Ding SQ. Acute pancreatitis: Etiology and common pathogenesis. World Journal of Gastroenterology. 2009;**15**(12):1427-1430

[7] Quinlan JD. Acute pancreatitis. American Family Physician. 2014;**90**(9):632-639

[8] Wu BU, Johannes RS, Sun X, et al. The early prediction of mortality in acute pancreatitis: a large population-based study. Gut 2008;**57**:1698.

[9] Banks PA, Bollen TL, Dervenis C, et al. Classification of acute pancreatitis—2012: Revision of the Atlanta classification and definitions by international consensus. Gut. 2013;**62**:102-111. DOI: 10.1136/gutjnl-2012-302779

[10] Ince AT, Baysal B. Pathophysiology, classification and available guidelines of acute Pancreatitis. The Turkish Journal of Gastroenterology. 2014;**25**:351-357

[11] Thoeni RF. The revised Atlanta classification of acute pancreatitis: Its importance for the radiologist and its effect on treatment. Radiology. 2012;**262**:751-764

[12] Suvarna R, Pallipady A, Bhandary N, Hanumanthappa. The clinical prognostic indicators of acute pancreatitis by Apac he II scoring. Journal of Clinical and Diagnostic Research. 2011;**5**(3):459-463

[13] Vincent JL, Abraham E, Moore FA, Kochanek PM, Fink MP. Text Book of Critical Care. 6th ed. Elsevier Saunders. Philadelphia, PA 19103-2899: 2011. pp. 804-813

[14] Bersten AD, Soni N. Oh's Intensive Care Manual. 6th ed. Butterwoth, Heinemann, Elsevier Oxford. pp. 479485

[15] Knaus WA, Draper EA, Wagner DP, Zimmerman JE (1985). "APACHE II: a severity of disease classification system". Critical Care Medicine. **13**(10):818-29.

[16] Sharma VK, Howden CW. Prophylactic antibiotic administration reduces sepsis and mortality in acute necrotizing pancreatitis: a meta-analysis. Pancreas 2001;**22**(1):28-31.

5

Current Neonatal Applications of Point-of-Care Ultrasound

Jae H. Kim, Nikolai Shalygin and Azif Safarulla

Abstract

Point-of-care ultrasound (POCUS) is an imaging modality that continues to gain acceptance in pediatric and neonatal medicine. In neonatology throughout many areas of the world, functional echocardiography performed by neonatologists has been at the forefront in the growth of POCUS compared to non-cardiac POCUS, the latter which potentially carries more opportunities for use. Despite the early adoption in obstetrics and maternal-fetal medicine, the actual bedside implementation in neonatology has unfortunately been much slower. Examples in neonatology where POCUS may continue to expand include central line placement, endotracheal tube localization, diagnosis of pneumothoraces, cardiac function assessment, and bowel viability assessment just to name a few. This chapter will be a practical synopsis of the most active uses and opportunities for POCUS in neonatology. Expanded training for neonatologists and trainees is required before widespread adoption occurs.

Keywords: ultrasound, point of care, newborn, preterm, central catheter, pneumothorax, necrotizing enterocolitis

1. Introduction

Point-of-care ultrasound (POCUS) is an imaging modality that continues to gain acceptance in pediatric and neonatal medicine. While ultrasound initially served as a clinical tool with a consultative model with radiology and cardiology disciplines, the value of POCUS in assessment of the heart and other organs is slowly being recognized. In neonatology throughout many areas of the world, functional echocardiography performed by neonatologists has been at the forefront in the growth of POCUS compared to non-cardiac POCUS. Technological advances have pushed ultrasound (US) to have improved image quality and mobility while reducing cost and size of devices increasing the availability of ultrasound as a point-of-care bedside tool in several areas such as emergency medicine, obstetrics, and intensive care. Despite the early adoption in obstetrics and maternal-fetal medicine, the actual bedside implementation in neonatology has unfortunately been much slower. Examples in neonatology where POCUS may continue to expand include central line placement, endotracheal tube localization, diagnosis of pneumothoraces, cardiac function assessment, and bowel viability assessment just to name a few. What follows is a practical synopsis of the most active uses and opportunities for POCUS in neonatology.

2. Head

The newborn brain is readily accessible for sonographic imaging by the open soft tissue windows of the anterior fontanelle and the open sutures found between the unfused cranial bones. Neonatologists are quite familiar with viewing and interpreting cranial ultrasound images as these are routinely reviewed daily on clinical rounds. The primary views are coronal (front to back), sagittal (left to right) and axial views for posterior fossa [1]. POCUS can provide excellent views of the general architecture of the brain especially the two ventricles, evaluation of hemorrhage or calcifications and early evidence of ischemic changes. The use of POCUS for brain imaging is particularly useful when suspect hemorrhage may be responsible for deterioration or hemodynamic instability, at times when sonographic support is not readily available. The detection of increased pressure, cerebral edema or stroke is not sensitive with HUS and other imaging modalities such as CT or MRI are recommended. It is important to remember that these evaluations are limited in evaluating this triangulated view of the brain and can miss events or lesions outside of this window in the parietal regions. Head ultrasound is one of the easier techniques to learn for neonatologists since the views are already very familiar to them. The imaging techniques hinge upon establishing stable upright views of the two hemispheres and axial views of the posterior fossa structures. Neonatal providers have ample experience in reviewing and interpreting head ultrasounds for common pathology such as periventricular leukomalacia, intraventricular and intracranial hemorrhages and so most of the skills are focused on imaging.

3. Central catheters

Central vascular catheters such as umbilical arterial catheters (UAC), umbilical venous catheters (UVC), and peripherally inserted central catheters (PICC) are the most common central catheters placed in the sick neonate. Any neonate born at less than 32 weeks gestation will have at least a UVC and/or a PICC during their admission for nutrition and/or medications. In most units all of these lines are placed blind and confirmed with a single radiograph. UVC tip localization by standard radiography is imprecise. In one study approximately 30% of the radiographs were read as normal but actually had the UVC tip in the right atrium when checked with US [2]. Radiographic localization of UVC on anterior–posterior (AP) is difficult to place in ideal position because of the doming of the diaphragm. The lateral chest radiograph is better than the AP view of the chest but this view is not as convenient with the infant typically secured down for the procedure.

Ultrasound more accurately confirms the position of the catheter tip than radiographs and reduces the exposure of ionizing radiation. Ultrasound guidance results in faster placement and fewer manipulations and radiographs for both umbilical catheters and PICC as compared with conventional placement [3, 4]. POCUS can be very useful in localizing the tip of central catheters either during placement or after a catheter has been placed to follow any migration. Umbilical catheters can frequently migrate after placement in the first few days after insertion. This may be due to drying and shrinkage of a longer umbilical cord. POCUS allows for the direct visualization of the umbilical and PICC catheters and their tips and indirect visualization of the UVC in the hepatic portion of the catheter pathway where it is localized by the shadow cast by the catheter [4]. Ultrasound may be able to help guide the catheter and thereby reduce complications during UVC, UAC, or PICC insertion. Doppler ultrasound is also useful to examine the aorta and renal vessels when placing or evaluating a UAC (**Figure 1**).

Use of POCUS for vascular access for PICCs has been limited due to the greater skillset required to accessing these small veins compared to older children. Setting up dedicated PICC teams can help develop this expertise to promote this aspect of central catheter POCUS.

With US, the UVC can be placed just beyond the IVC-RA junction. This permits good visualization and eliminates any risk of extravasation of the catheter in the liver. The UAC is readily placed just behind the heart which approximates the T7–8 position. The recognition of PICC movement in the large vessels makes it particularly challenging to manage the best position to place these catheters. Movement of the arm or leg to identify the deepest position of the PICC will ensure that the catheter does not inadvertently migrate deeper after placement and cause more risk of complications. For upper PICCs the arm position in a 45 degree flexed position at the shoulder and elbow usually represents the deepest point for a PICC while the knees bent close to the chest represent the deepest point for lower PICCs. The upper PICC can be placed at least 1 cm before the SVC-RA junction while the lower PICC is placed at 1–2 cm below the IVC-RA junction (**Figure 2**).

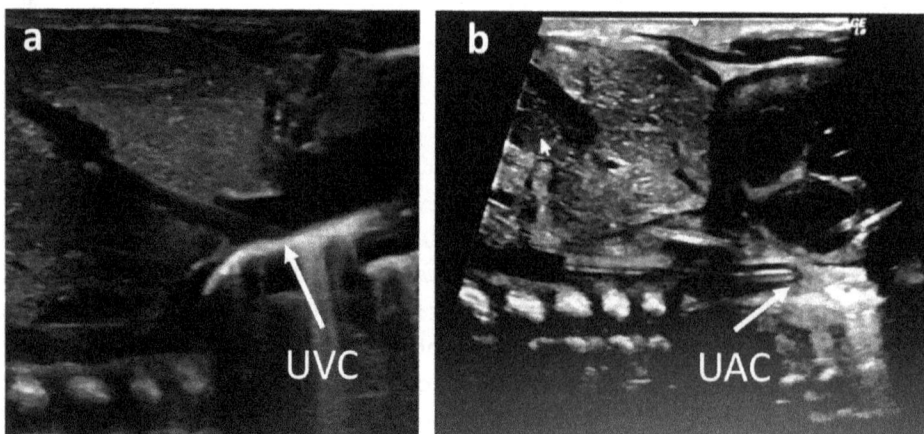

Figure 1. Umbilical catheter placement (a) UVC-umbilical venous catheter, (b) UAC-umbilical arterial catheter.

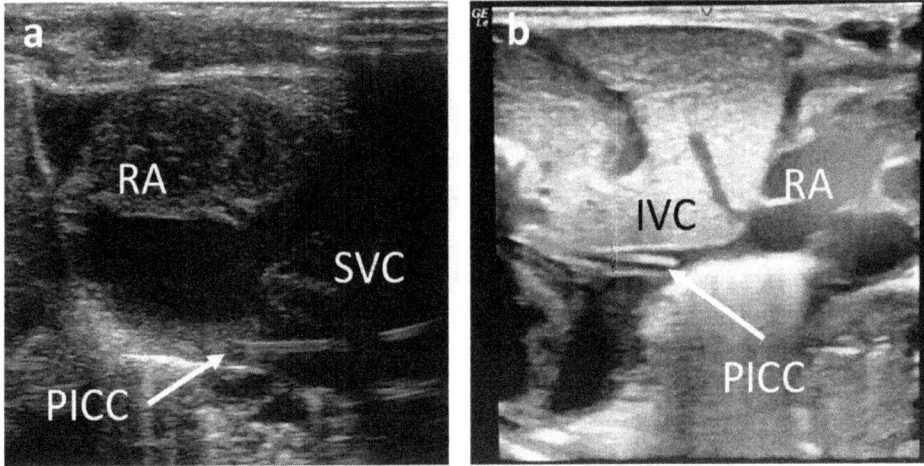

Figure 2. PICC localization (a) upper PICC, (b) lower PICC, PICC-peripherally, inserted central catheter, RA-right atrium, SVC-superior vena cava, IVC-inferior vena cava.

Other areas of benefit from POCUS in the NICU are arterial line placement where localization of the vessel and flow identification by Doppler ultrasound can be performed. A modified Allen test with Doppler ultrasound evaluation of collateral flow is useful prior to the procedure. Real-time ultrasound can result in fewer attempts and less chance of a hematoma as compared with palpation.

4. Cardiac

The use of echocardiography has aided the evaluation of cardiac anatomy and function of the unborn fetus and the newborn. Ordering an assessment of the heart by ultrasound is a routine practice in the NICU. There has been a need to supplement the clinical assessment and current hemodynamic monitoring as they do not provide a comprehensive picture of cardiac output and organ perfusion states. The need for serial measurements is another unmet need with routine cardiac echocardiograms since transitional physiology after birth and during illness often require repeated measurements. Bedside POCUS for cardiac assessment is still an emerging practice as training to evaluate the heart is one of the hardest POCUS skills. Despite its difficulty there are probably more neonatologists worldwide with training to assess the heart through limited functional assessments than there are for non-cardiac POCUS. Cardiac POCUS is not intended to replace a cardiology assessment or structural echocardiogram. It is intended to be limited and dynamic assessment of hemodynamic of the heart to help with clinical decision making. Cardiac assessment in neonates is unique due to the dynamic changes that occur in the first few weeks of life making it challenging to order frequent dynamic assessments. The ability to help determine rapid determination of hemodynamics with serial functional assessments makes it increasingly attractive to work it into the daily workflow [5]. The focus of neonatal cardiac POCUS is to concentrate on a limited set of assessments that are helpful in determining the real-time hemodynamics. These include assessment of the patent ductus arteriosus (PDA), ventricular function, filling of the heart and volume assessment.

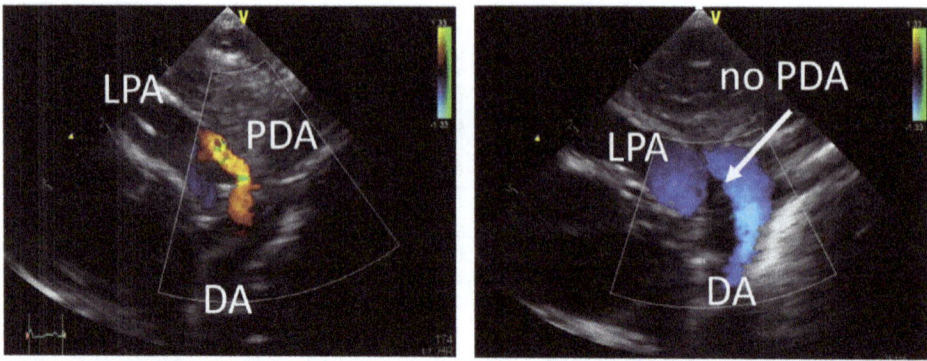

Figure 3. PDA (a) large PDA, (b) no PDA, LPA-left pulmonary artery, DA-descending aorta.

To start, cardiac POCUS can provide a rapid qualitative assessment of contractility: normal, hyperactive, reduced contractility (mild, moderate, or severe). Fractional shortening measurements are relatively easy to obtain and provide quantitative information. Cardiac filling as a measure of volume assessment can also be determined quickly. The PDA represents an important shunt to assess to facilitate clinical management to determine if the PDA is contributing to cardiorespiratory compromise or systemic hypoperfusion. The PDA can be determined to be open or closed (**Figure 3**). The presence of a patent ductus arteriosus can lead to an overestimate of cardiac output using usual left ventricular output measurements. An alternative measure of cardiac output using superior vena caval flow (SVC) measurements as a surrogate measure has been proposed [6–9]. Unfortunately, SVC flow has not become widely used as it has proven to be difficult to minimize inter-operator variability in this measurement. While several examples of benefit of neonatal cardiac POCUS have been published, there remains a paucity of neonatal clinical studies to validate each of the functional assessments and their ability to improve diagnostic or management of the sick neonate [10, 11]. As more neonatologists become comfortable with the skillset of cardiac echocardiography, there is a need for improved standardization and quality assurance [12, 13]. There have been some attempt to standardize the practice but many feel that the standards set are excessive and restrict early adoption [14, 15]. The anatomic assessment of the heart for the most part should be left to the cardiologist but it is equally important to recognize patterns of normal structure to know when there is suspicion of a congenital heart lesion.

Nevertheless, despite a number of hurdles, there remains tremendous promise that neonatal cardiac POCUS can provide a focused assessment to provide hemodynamic information to the bedside clinician.

5. Lung

The evaluation of lung by POCUS in neonates is increasingly practiced as the imaging technique is relatively simple and the lung is readily accessible for interrogation through the chest wall. Several recent articles have noted lung ultrasound to be as good if not better than X-ray as a diagnostic modality. Reduction in cost of image acquisition and exposure to ionizing radiation improves quality of care as well as patient safety [16]. Neonatal lung POCUS is similar to pediatric lung POCUS except that the neonate has very thin soft tissue in the chest with thin ribs and a cartilaginous sternum that enables larger windows of viewing. From a technical perspective, we need a high frequency transducer like a 7–15 MHz hockey stick or equivalent linear array transducer. The detection of common respiratory conditions has been documented making it potentially possible to define the parenchymal lung disease by characteristic patterns to the common respiratory conditions such as pneumonia (PNA), transient tachypnea of the newborn (TTN) and respiratory distress syndrome (RDS). The ability to make an urgent diagnosis is where the greatest utility of lung POCUS may lie as acute respiratory compromise often requires rapid diagnostics. The presence of air or fluid such as blood, transudate or exudate in the pleural space is readily discernable by US.

The complication of spontaneous pneumothorax (PTX) at birth is one such condition that may be aided by lung POCUS. PTX will display several differing US patterns compared to normal lung. The characteristic findings on US of PTX in neonates are similar to adults and children (**Figure 4**). Normal lung appears homogeneous in texture with the occasional presence of hyperechoic linear A (horizontal) and B (vertical) lines. Movement of the parietal and visceral pleura against each other during respiration creates a "shimmering effect" or an "ants marching effect" which is termed lung sliding. The presence of the sliding lung sign rules out a pneumothorax on B mode [17]. Further confirmation of a PTX can be achieved with M mode which displays the data from a single line in an image mapped against time on the x-axis. The appearance of moving lung tissue results in a granular appearance similar to a sandy "seashore" with the "waves" at the top representing the static soft tissue above the lungs. Some data suggests that US may not be as sensitive for PTX in neonates [18].

The underlying changes in RDS involve loss of the smallest airspaces (alveoli or saccules). This generates denser tissue that gives the appearance of "white lung" using lung POCUS. Some have proposed a scoring system to categorize lung disease in RDS to assist in increasing specificity for diagnosing RDS [19]. This score can reliably predict the need for surfactant treatment in preterm babies less than 34 weeks gestation treated with nasal CPAP from birth. Several

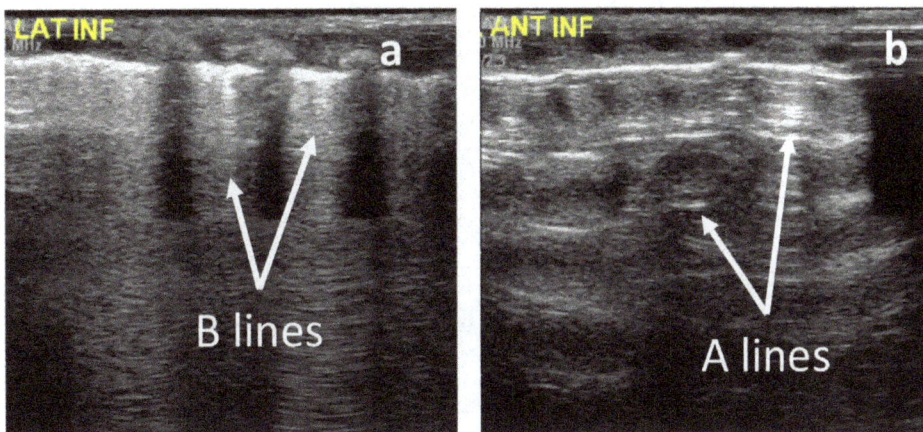

Figure 4. Pneumothorax (a) normal lung, (b) pneumothorax.

studies have validated the ability to distinguish between RDS and transient tachypnea of the newborn (TTN) [20, 21]. In TTN ultrasound changes include abnormalities of pleural lines, absence of A-lines, and interstitial syndrome or pulmonary edema. Pneumonia has been described to have A-lines, interstitial syndrome and possible lung consolidation. Lung POCUS has been able to differentiate meconium aspiration syndrome from other respiratory conditions since it is also associated with absent A-lines, lung consolidation, and interstitial syndrome.

The role of lung ultrasound may not replace chest radiographs but may offer more time sensitive information and reduce the total number of radiographs taken. The evaluation of lung by POCUS in neonates is increasingly being studied and practiced. The most promising application may be during resuscitation where early detection and management of conditions like pneumothoraces and pleural effusions are life-saving.

6. Endotracheal tube

Neonatal intubation remains a difficult high level skill. Although there are much less intubations taking place compared to a decade ago, the need to establish a secure airway remains ever important. This is particularly true for resuscitation of neonates <28 weeks gestation. The current standard of practice to confirm the placement of the endotracheal tube (ETT) is with chest x-ray (CXR).The passage of the ETT into the trachea or esophagus can be discerned readily using a transverse probe position in adults and pediatric subjects [22–25]. POCUS can be used to rapidly and accurately visualize the anatomic position of the ETT position in preterm and term infants [26] (**Figure 5**). Unlike in pediatric or adult patients, evaluating the ETT in the newborn

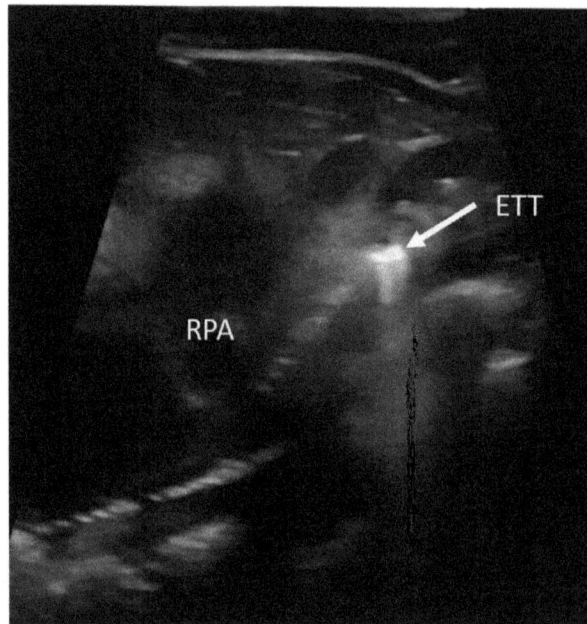

Figure 5. Endotracheal tube placement ETT-endotracheal tube, RPA-right pulmonary artery.

through the chest is possible due to the cartilaginous sternum. Although there is air inside and around the ETT and the entry is at a steep angle to the ultrasound probe, the tip of the probe can be identified with a white or hyperechoic line. The ideal location for the tip of the ETT is midway between the thoracic inlet and the carina. Identifying the distance of the tip of the ETT from the carina can be accurately measured. In a recent publication of an extensive database literature search on studies relating to US use for ETT position confirmation found nine studies which collectively reported a > 80% visualization of the ETT tip by US [22]. Also, US interpretation of the ETT position correlated with the XR position in 73–100% of cases. US appears comparable to XR determining ETT position in this population. As US is more easily available and is safer than CXR, it may be a better modality for confirming proper placement of ETT in neonates when time is critical. There are no current data yet on identifying tip location during placement of the ETT and so more clinical data may be required before widespread adoption.

7. Bowel

The assessment of bowel by POCUS in neonates remains an emerging practice despite the availability of clinical data in neonates for more than a decade. POCUS can show dynamic intestinal peristalsis as well as characterize the physical nature and perfusion of bowel that can be used to assess bowel integrity and viability. The newborn can be affected by a variety of congenital and acquired bowel conditions that may lead to significant bowel dysfunction or even death. Early recognition of the signs of impending bowel injury or the progression of bowel damage is essential. Intestinal peristalsis can be quantified by counting cumulative motility events over time to give an objective assessment of bowel movement [27]. Identifying peristalsis can assist in the routine management of neonatal feeding or bowel assessment but more studies are required to validate its utility for clinical outcomes (**Figure 6**). Some other studies have demonstrated that gastroesophageal reflux can be evaluated by POCUS both identifying anatomic risk factors as well as visualizing the bolus but this has not gained traction in clinical practice yet [28, 29].

Recent data suggest that dedicated abdominal ultrasound examination may be of utility in the diagnosis and management of infants with necrotizing enterocolitis (NEC). Advantages of ultrasound include assessment of peristalsis, vascular perfusion, bowel-wall thickening, and abdominal fluid. Absence of ionizing radiation is an added benefit. A recent meta-analysis showed that bowel ultrasound is increasingly being recognized as an important imaging tool for evaluating NEC that provides additional detail over plain abdominal radiographs [30]. There are still only few studies with small case series and heterogeneous gestational age population that have investigated the comparison between plain radiographs and abdominal ultrasound in predicting the outcomes of patients with NEC.

NEC is one of the most severe gastrointestinal conditions affecting neonates. The risk increases with degree of prematurity and in those with low birth weight [31–35]. Although risk factors have been identified, the etiology is still not well recognized. Despite significant advances in neonatal care, mortality in NEC remains high (between 20 and 60% in a group of most immature neonates) and maintained at the same level. Therefore, in cases of clinically suspected

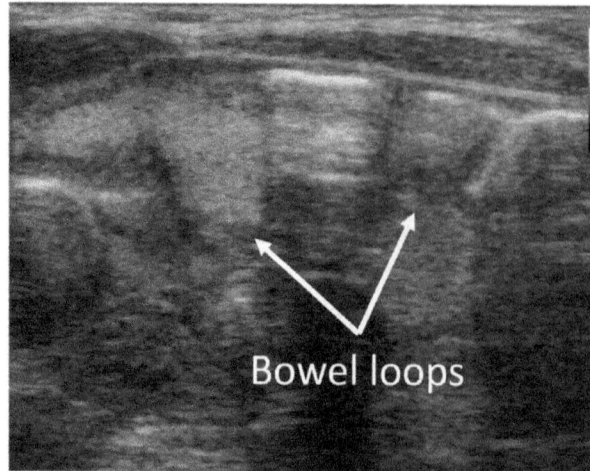

Figure 6. Normal bowel appearance.

NEC quick diagnostics and implementation of appropriate treatment are crucial [34–36]. Diagnosis is based on clinical presentation, laboratory testing and imaging. Traditionally, the gold standard for imaging evaluation of the neonatal intestine is the intestinal gas pattern on plain abdominal radiographs; however interpretation can be challenging with intestinal gas pattern being nonspecific [37–39], and significant overlap between radiographic signs of NEC and other intestinal pathology [40].

The usefulness of abdominal ultrasound in the diagnosis of NEC has been known since 1984 as evidenced in a number of studies [41–43]. Studies have looked at ultrasound being an adjunct to diagnose and manage infants with NEC. It allows for an earlier detection of typical signs of NEC, with more rapid disease management. When compared with abdominal radiographs in predicting NEC, studies showed that they can depict bowel distension, to some extent bowel-wall thickness, pneumatosis intestinalis, portal venous air and free abdominal air which ultrasound could easily depict as well. More importantly, abdominal ultrasound provides important additional information regarding viability of bowel wall viability and free fluid, which might aid in diagnosis and management of NEC [44, 45]. With color Doppler specific suspicious loops of bowel can be interrogated to reveal if they are perfused or not which enables the identification of non-viable bowel with a high degree of certainty. The gradual progression of NEC can be identified by POCUS from the initial hyperemia and swelling of bowel wall to the dilatation with increased disease and then thinning of bowel wall with loss of perfusion or blood flow. Therefore, nonviable bowel will no longer have any blood flow present (**Figure 7 Epelman diagram**). The detection of portal venous gas is much easier by POCUS than by radiographs [46].

7.1. Procedure and features

For performing bowel ultrasound a linear probe of 8–15 MHz probe (higher frequency for higher resolution and lower depth targeting superficial structures). Features that are key include: (a) bowel wall thickening >2.6 mm, (b) increase in bowel wall echogenicity, (c) portal venous air, (d) pneumatosis Intestinalis and free air and (e) intra-abdominal fluid.

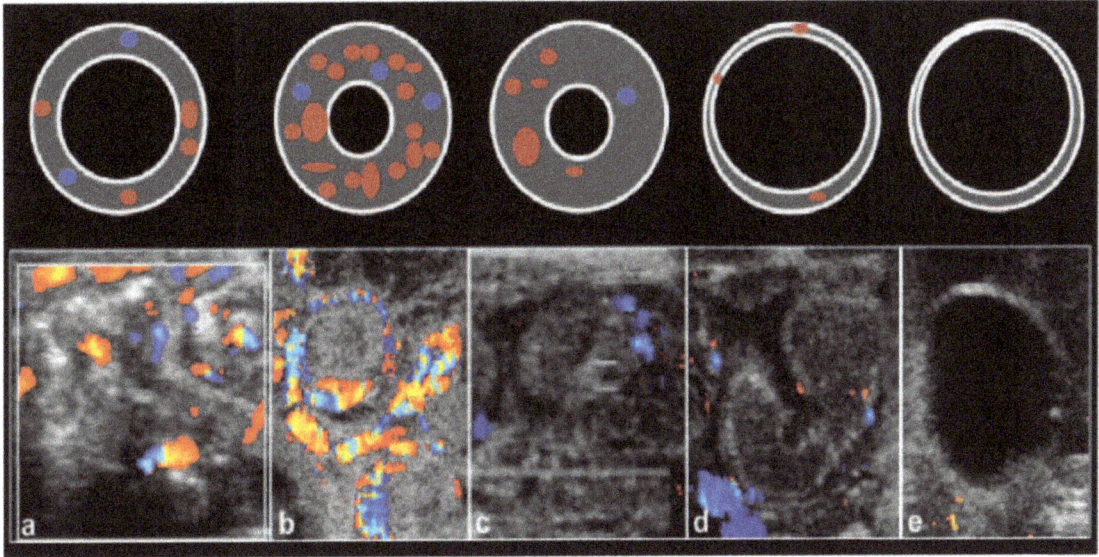

Figure 7. Sonographic appearance of NEC progression (figure from Epelman et al. 38 need permission).

Some limitations of ultrasound include that it is operator or skill dependent and this is a real time diagnosis which might create an obstacle for radiologists to evaluate the ultrasounds retrospectively and in turn underlines the need for neonatologists to be more familiar with this tool. Currently most of the available literature are single center trials, retrospective observational cohorts. We still need more prospective studies doing head to head trials with abdominal radiograph to understand the true value and usefulness of abdominal US. More studies are required to fully validate these assessments in clinical care. Training of radiologist and their sonographers as well as other providers such as neonatologists and surgeons is required before broad adoption of bowel POCUS occurs.

8. Bladder

Bladder aspiration through suprapubic urine collection is ideal to perform under ultrasound guidance over landmark techniques. Ultrasound of the bladder can help determine the size and location of the bladder and the volume of urine in the bladder. Portable ultrasound can significantly improve the diagnostic yield; a minimum volume on ultrasound of 10 mL is associated with a 90% successful bladder aspiration. If the cephalocaudal diameter of the bladder (sagittal view) is >20 mm and the anteroposterior diameter is >15 mm, the success rate approaches 100%.

9. Lumbar puncture

Lumbar puncture (LP) is a relatively common procedure performed in emergency department and the NICU as part of a complete sepsis evaluation. The LP is typically performed using the "blind" surface landmark guidance. Anecdotally, this technique is reported to be have a high percentage of success. However successful identification of landmarks has been shown to be accurate only 30% of the time [47]. Traumatic or unsuccessful LPs in this group have been documented in the pediatric literature in 30–50% of patients [48, 49]. This translates to increased difficulty in obtaining CSF and higher rate of complications such as local/subdural/epidural hematoma, bloody tap and incomplete sepsis evaluation to name a few. Fluoroscopy guided LP is an alternative but challenges include limited availability, radiation exposure, need to transport critical patients for the procedure.

Use of POCUS for identification of key landmarks is a safe and easy alternative to the blind method [50–52]. In adults, using ultrasound for LP has been associated with a reduction in the number of attempts and interspaces accessed [51–55]. In neonates, the incompletely ossified spinous processes, minimal fat aids in interrogation of the space by ultrasound compared to older kids and adults. The good resolution of image, lack of ionizing radiation and potential for real time guidance makes ultrasound a valuable tool for performing LP in neonates [48, 56].

LP can be performed in the neonate without general anesthesia or sedation, using oral sucrose and local anesthesia. Patient can be in lateral decubitus position or sitting up. Using ultrasound to measure the interspinous space at L3-L4 and L4-L5 in varying positions, the lumbar spine is found to be maximally positioned in both neonates and children in the seated position with flexed hips versus the lateral decubitus position [57, 58]. The probe used is the 7–15 MHz hockey stick or equivalent linear array transducer. There is still very limited knowledge on ultrasound guided LP in neonates. There are two techniques described in literature, the transverse approach and longitudinal approach based on how the probe is held.

The first skill is to define the landmarks for the LP procedure. Using a surgical marker or pen one can delineate the location of midline and the position of the conus, the point where the spinal cord ends. There are no studies validating the guidance of the needle into the interspace and so this will require more studies before guidance by US is a routine procedure.

10. Summary

Existing and emerging POCUS applications are numerous and promising but more validation for clinical value is required in addition to larger scale training of individuals to learn and become competent in these techniques. Emphasis should be on training all incoming and existing fellows to learn POCUS.

Author details

Jae H. Kim[1]*, Nikolai Shalygin[1] and Azif Safarulla[2]

*Address all correspondence to: neojae@ucsd.edu

1 University of California San Diego and Rady Children's Hospital of San Diego, San Diego, California, USA

2 Augusta University, Augusta, Georgia, USA

References

[1] Bhat V, Bhat V. Neonatal neurosonography: A pictorial essay. Indian Journal of Radiology Imaging. 2014;**24**(4):389-400

[2] Karber BC et al. Optimal radiologic position of an umbilical venous catheter tip as determined by echocardiography in very low birth weight newborns. Journal of Neonatal-Perinatal Medicine. 2017;**10**(1):55-61

[3] Katheria AC, Fleming SE, Kim JH. A randomized controlled trial of ultrasound-guided peripherally inserted central catheters compared with standard radiograph in neonates. Journal of Perinatology. 2013;**33**(10):791-794

[4] Fleming SE, Kim JH. Ultrasound-guided umbilical catheter insertion in neonates. Journal of Perinatology. 2011;**31**(5):344-349

[5] Poon WB, Wong KY. Neonatologist-performed point-of-care functional echocardiography in the neonatal intensive care unit. Singapore Medical Journal. 2017;**58**(5):230-233

[6] Evans N. Diagnosis of the preterm patent ductus arteriosus: Clinical signs, biomarkers, or ultrasound? Seminars in Perinatology. 2012;**36**(2):114-122

[7] Kluckow M, Seri I, Evans N. Echocardiography and the neonatologist. Pediatric Cardiology. 2008;**29**(6):1043-1047

[8] Kluckow M, Evans N. Low superior vena cava flow and intraventricular haemorrhage in preterm infants. Archives of Disease in Childhood. Fetal and Neonatal Edition. 2000;**82**(3):F188-F194

[9] Kluckow M, Evans N. Superior vena cava flow in newborn infants: A novel marker of systemic blood flow. Archives of Disease in Childhood. Fetal and Neonatal Edition. 2000;**82**(3):F182-F187

[10] Sehgal A, Paul E, Menahem S. Functional echocardiography in staging for ductal disease severity: Role in predicting outcomes. European Journal of Pediatrics. 2013;**172**(2):179-184

[11] Sehgal A, McNamara PJ. Does echocardiography facilitate determination of hemodynamic significance attributable to the ductus arteriosus? European Journal of Pediatrics. 2009;**168**(8):907-914

[12] Finan E et al. Targeted neonatal echocardiography services: Need for standardized training and quality assurance. Journal of Ultrasound in Medicine. 2014;**33**(10):1833-1841

[13] Lee HC, Silverman N, Hintz SR. Diagnosis of patent ductus arteriosus by a neonatologist with a compact, portable ultrasound machine. Journal of Perinatology. 2007;**27**(5):291-296

[14] Mertens L et al. Targeted neonatal echocardiography in the neonatal intensive care unit: Practice guidelines and recommendations for training: Writing group of the American Society of Echocardiography (ASE) in collaboration with the European Association

of Echocardiography (EAE) and the Association for European Pediatric Cardiologists (AEPC). European Journal of Echocardiography. 2011;**12**(10):715-736

[15] Singh Y et al. Expert consensus statement 'Neonatologist-performed echocardiography (NoPE)'-training and accreditation in UK. European Journal of Pediatrics. 2016; **175**(2):281-287

[16] Hall EJ. Lessons we have learned from our children: Cancer risks from diagnostic radiology. Pediatric Radiology. 2002;**32**(10):700-706

[17] Kurepa D, Zaghloul N, Watkins L, Liu J. Neonatal lung ultrasound exam guidelines. Journal of Perinatology. 2018 Jan;**38**(1):11-22

[18] Liu DM et al. Utilization of ultrasound for the detection of pneumothorax in the neonatal special-care nursery. Pediatric Radiology. 2003;**33**(12):880-883

[19] Brat R et al. Lung ultrasonography score to evaluate oxygenation and surfactant need in neonates treated with continuous positive airway pressure. JAMA Pediatrics. 2015; **169**(8):e151797

[20] Liu J et al. Lung ultrasonography to diagnose transient tachypnea of the newborn. Chest. 2016;**149**(5):1269-1275

[21] Sawires HK et al. Use of lung ultrasound in detection of complications of respiratory distress syndrome. Ultrasound in Medicine & Biology. 2015;**41**(9):2319-2325

[22] Jaeel P, Sheth M, Nguyen J. Ultrasonography for endotracheal tube position in infants and children. European Journal of Pediatrics. 2017;**176**(3):293-300

[23] Slovis TL, Poland RL. Endotracheal tubes in neonates: Sonographic positioning. Radiology. 1986;**160**(1):262-263

[24] Sethi A et al. Point of care ultrasonography for position of tip of endotracheal tube in neonates. Indian Pediatrics. 2014;**51**(2):119-121

[25] Tejesh CA et al. Sonographic detection of tracheal or esophageal intubation: A cadaver study. Saudi Journal of Anaesthesia. 2016;**10**(3):314-316

[26] Dennington D et al. Ultrasound confirmation of endotracheal tube position in neonates. Neonatology. 2012;**102**(3):185-189

[27] Richburg DA, Kim JH. Real-time bowel ultrasound to characterize intestinal motility in the preterm neonate. Journal of Perinatology. 2013;**33**(8):605-608

[28] Pezzati M et al. Diagnosis of gastro-oesophageal reflux in preterm infants: Sonography vs. pH-monitoring. Neonatology. 2007;**91**(3):162-166

[29] Koumanidou C et al. Sonographic measurement of the abdominal esophagus length in infancy: A diagnostic tool for gastroesophageal reflux. AJR. American Journal of Roentgenology. 2004;**183**(3):801-807

[30] Cuna AC et al. Bowel ultrasound for predicting surgical management of necrotizing entero-colitis: A systematic review and meta-analysis. Pediatric Radiology. 2017;**48**(5):658-666

[31] Schnabl KL et al. Necrotizing enterocolitis: A multifactorial disease with no cure. World Journal of Gastroenterology. 2008;**14**(14):2142-2161

[32] Neu J, Walker WA. Necrotizing enterocolitis. The New England Journal of Medicine. 2011;**364**(3):255-264

[33] Lin PW, Stoll BJ. Necrotising enterocolitis. Lancet. 2006;**368**(9543):1271-1283

[34] Holman RC et al. Necrotising enterocolitis hospitalisations among neonates in the United States. Paediatric and Perinatal Epidemiology. 2006;**20**(6):498-506

[35] Clark RH et al. Characteristics of patients who die of necrotizing enterocolitis. Journal of Perinatology. 2012;**32**(3):199-204

[36] Luig M et al. Epidemiology of necrotizing enterocolitis–part II: Risks and susceptibility of premature infants during the surfactant era: A regional study. Journal of Paediatrics and Child Health. 2005;**41**(4):174-179

[37] Rehan VK et al. Observer variability in interpretation of abdominal radiographs of infants with suspected necrotizing enterocolitis. Clinical Pediatrics (Phila). 1999;**38**(11):637-643

[38] Baird R et al. Imaging, radiation exposure, and attributable cancer risk for neonates with necrotizing enterocolitis. Journal of Pediatric Surgery. 2013;**48**(5):1000-1005

[39] Coursey CA et al. Radiologists' agreement when using a 10-point scale to report abdomi-nal radiographic findings of necrotizing enterocolitis in neonates and infants. American Journal of Roentgenology. 2008;**191**(1):190-197

[40] Epelman M et al. Necrotizing enterocolitis: Review of state-of-the-art imaging findings with pathologic correlation. Radiographics. 2007;**27**(2):285-305

[41] Yikilmaz A et al. Prospective evaluation of the impact of sonography on the manage-ment and surgical intervention of neonates with necrotizing enterocolitis. Pediatric Surgery International. 2014;**30**(12):1231-1240

[42] Raboisson MJ et al. Assessment of uterine artery and aortic isthmus Doppler record-ings as predictors of necrotizing enterocolitis. American Journal of Obstetrics and Gynecology. 2012;**206**(3): 232 e1-6

[43] Akin MA et al. Quantitative assessment of hepatic blood flow in the diagnosis and management of necrotizing enterocolitis. The Journal of Maternal-Fetal & Neonatal Medicine. 2015;**28**(18):2160-2165

[44] Higashizono K et al. Postoperative pneumatosis intestinalis (PI) and portal venous gas (PVG) may indicate bowel necrosis: A 52-case study. BMC Surgery. 2016;**16**(1):42

[45] Nevins EJ et al. A rare case of ischaemic pneumatosis intestinalis and hepatic portal venous gas in an elderly patient with good outcome following conservative manage-ment. International Journal of Surgery Case Reports. 2016;**25**:167-170

[46] Bohnhorst B et al. Early feeding after necrotizing enterocolitis in preterm infants. The Journal of Pediatrics. 2003;**143**(4):484-487

[47] Furness G, Reilly MP, Kuchi S. An evaluation of ultrasound imaging for identification of lumbar intervertebral level. Anaesthesia. 2002;**57**(3):277-280

[48] Coley BD, Shiels WE 2nd, Hogan MJ. Diagnostic and interventional ultrasonography in neonatal and infant lumbar puncture. Pediatric Radiology. 2001;**31**(6):399-402

[49] Glatstein MM et al. Incidence of traumatic lumbar puncture: Experience of a large, tertiary care pediatric hospital. Clinical Pediatrics (Phila). 2011;**50**(11):1005-1009

[50] Dietrich AM, Coley BD. Bedside pediatric emergency evaluation through ultrasonography. Pediatric Radiology. 2008;**38**(Suppl 4):S679-S684

[51] Ozdamar E et al. Ultrasound-assisted lumbar puncture in pediatric emergency department. Pediatric Emergency Care. 2017;**33**(8):e21-e23

[52] Nomura JT et al. A randomized controlled trial of ultrasound-assisted lumbar puncture. Journal of Ultrasound in Medicine. 2007;**26**(10):1341-1348

[53] Brousseau AA, Parent MC. Towards evidence based emergency medicine: Best BETs from the Manchester Royal Infirmary. BET 3: Advantages of ultrasound-assisted lumbar puncture. Emergency Medicine Journal. 2016;**33**(2):163-165

[54] Strony R. Ultrasound-assisted lumbar puncture in obese patients. Critical Care Clinics. 2010;**26**(4):661-664

[55] Shaikh F et al. Ultrasound imaging for lumbar punctures and epidural catheterisations: Systematic review and meta-analysis. BMJ. 2013;**346**:f1720

[56] Abukawa Y et al. Ultrasound versus anatomical landmarks for caudal epidural anesthesia in pediatric patients. BMC Anesthesiology. 2015;**15**:102

[57] Abo A et al. Positioning for lumbar puncture in children evaluated by bedside ultrasound. Pediatrics. 2010;**125**(5):e1149-e1153

[58] Oncel S et al. Positioning of infants in the neonatal intensive care unit for lumbar puncture as determined by bedside ultrasonography. Archives of Disease in Childhood. Fetal and Neonatal Edition. 2013;**98**(2):F133-F135

6

Intensive Care Unit Workforce: Occupational Health and Safety

Melek Nihal Esin and Duygu Sezgin

Abstract

There are many different work tasks and workplace hazards related to the ICU setting. The workplace hazards include the physical environment of the ICU, working conditions, psychosocial factors, ergonomic factors, biological factors and chemical factors that cause ICU workers to have health problems. The occurrence of occupational health problems in ICU workers not only leads to decreased job satisfaction and productivity but also increases absenteeism and burnout. Moreover, this situation adversely affects patient care and increases the cost of treatment. Recognising occupational hazards and risks arising from the work environment will assist in planning strategies to protect and promote health programmes for ICU workers. Understanding the importance of occupational health and safety practices by all institutions is a key factor to improve quality of life, work efficiency and work satisfaction of ICU workers.

Keywords: intensive care unit, ICU workforce, workplace hazards, occupational health, occupational safety

1. Introduction

This chapter presents information about occupational health and safety in the intensive care unit (ICU) settings. The reader is cautioned that ICU workers face many workplace hazards due to the complex nature of their work environment. Furthermore, this chapter aims to describe the occupational risks of ICU workers related to personal factors and to discuss prevention strategies related to this issue. Although traditional prevention strategies for occupational health and safety in the ICU are given, personal measures such as risk management and health promotion programmes for ICU workforce will also be provided.

2. Intensive care unit workforce

The health services provided in ICUs are carried out by a multidisciplinary team. The members of this team are intensivists, ICU nurses, pharmacists, dieticians, respiratory therapists, physiotherapists, occupational therapists, healthcare assistants and members of other professions [1, 2]. Other staff in secretarial and transportation services are in a position to support the ICU team [2].

The nursing staff in some countries may comprise distinct occupations such as nurses and nurse aids/assistants or technicians [3]. Nurses are the workforce in the ICU and are mostly involved in complex work tasks, such as medication management, organising the ICU environment, coordinating the work tasks between nursing staff and direct contact with patients while providing care, as well [3]. The working experience of the ICU nursing staff may vary with the hospital type and location. In the study done by Sevinç et al. [5], 30% of the ICU nurses had working experience of less than 1 year. In another study setting done in the United States, the mean age of ICU nurses was 46.5 [7]. Healthcare assistants are responsible for tasks related to patient care directly, inasmuch as they are the members of the ICU team that are most exposed to the physical workloads [3].

The work environment in the ICU setting poses many occupational hazards, especially for the female workforce. In recent years, the number of female intensive care medicine (ICM) specialists has increased. Studies show that the proportion of female ICM specialists in the United Kingdom and New Zealand in 2012 was 17% and 18%, respectively. On the other hand, majority of the nursing workforce in the ICUs consists of women. Although the nursing profession has become more popular for men in the recent years, female nurses in the clinical setting still have a slightly higher percentage than male nurses. Thus, the occupational hazards and challenges for female members of the ICU team must be considered during the risk assessment, hazard prevention and training processes as they might face higher risks due to pregnancy, motherhood and other conditions) [4].

Due to the fact that working conditions are hazardous in the ICU setting, nurses and other ICU workers transfer to other units in the hospitals after working there for a certain period. As in many other units in the hospitals, there are also shortages of staff in the ICU setting. Many studies show that inadequate numbers of the ICU staff have a negative impact on patient outcomes [5, 6]. However, not only the number of staff will prevent unexpected negative conditions of the patients, but also the work environment will improve patient outcomes [7].

The models advocating the improvement of patient outcomes and cost-effectiveness support having an intensivist present in the ICU setting, creating accurate job descriptions for all team members, developing procedures and providing continuous education to the staff [2].

3. The work environment in the ICU and the occupational hazards

The work environment is considered an important factor that affects the motivation and work satisfaction of employees. A productive and satisfying work environment is described as *"a multi-dimensional, integrated phenomenon"* and the importance of having all dimensions present in the work setting is stated by Schmalenberg and Kramer as *"an excellent work environment doesn't evolve from the presence of only a few desired processes. None of them optional, all are required."* [8].

The workplace environment must be considered carefully because of the fact that it can affect the motivation and capability of ICU workers to perform the tasks [9]. There is evidence about the impact of poor work environments on healthcare professionals and patient outcomes [7]. Negative outcomes for the ICU workforce can be related to job satisfaction and burnout. However, there are some other negative outcomes for the patients such as inadequate safety, impaired quality of care, medical errors and increased mortality [7].

The work environment in ICU is not only related to the physical environment, but also related to psychosocial settings [7]. The nature of a poor work environment is associated with a number of hazards and risks [10]. The terms "hazard" and "risk" are often used interchangeably which leads to confusion. Despite this, hazards in the workplace are described as "a potential source of harm or adverse health effect on a person or persons" [11, 12]. Additionally, the risks which arise from identified hazards are graded by combinations of severity and likelihood of harm [11, 13].

The ICU environment may cause a number of health risks in relation to occupational hazards. The workplace hazards include the **physical environment** of the ICU (*lighting, conditioning, noise, equipment, work space*), **working conditions** (*daily workload, working in shifts, standing for long hours, caring for patients with co-morbidities, inadequate income*), **psychosocial factors** (*dissatisfaction with work, workplace stress, frequently encountered deaths, interaction with families of patients, workplace violence*), **ergonomic factors** (*repositioning the patients* and *repeating movements such as pushing, pulling, elevating* and *bending*), **biological factors** (*being exposed to infectious organisms during invasive and non-invasive procedures*) and **chemical factors** (*being exposed to antiseptic and disinfectants or inhaling their gases*).

3.1. Physical environment

The physical environment of the ICU may contain various hazards likely to cause injuries to ICU workers. Those hazards are associated with mechanical factors, equipment, noise, light, heat and humidity. In the conditions where the physical characteristics of the workplace were not designed considering the needs and expectations of employees, it will result in decreased work performance of the employees and increased number of lost work days [14].

Mechanical hazards in the ICU include mobile equipment which is used to transfer patients, transported objects i.e. emergency trolleys, moving parts of objects, sharp edges of surfaces, falling objects, slippery surfaces, high pressure fluids and other items. ICU staff are more likely to sustain injuries caused by mechanical hazards inasmuch as they give care to patients in unstable conditions. A suitable workplace design, safety signs and risk measures should be applied to eliminate risks related to mechanical hazards in the ICU [15].

Intensive care units are one of the departments with the most advanced equipment in the hospital settings. With the aim of using that equipment effectively, it is important to design the bed spaces, monitor heights and drainage systems considering the architectural principles for the ICU standards so that healthcare personnel can have sufficient space to care for their patients [16, 17]. The environment of the ICU requires appropriate physical layout and workstation design. On the other hand, an inadequate patient room or bed space will make it difficult to interact effectively with the patient and provided equipment [9]. The architectural design of the ICU affects job satisfaction, the level of stress and well-being of the healthcare professionals working in the ICU setting. The ICU team members' experiences and opinions should be asked for before the architectural design of the ICU is made [17].

The equipment to improve the physical conditions might not have been developed yet for the specific needs in the ICU; on the other hand, it might be developed but not obtained by the facility (the hospital) or provided in some ICU setting [9]. The studies show that although in some ICU setting the staff are provided high technological equipment to prevent them from physical injuries and protect them from musculoskeletal disorders, they do not make use of the equipment reporting reasons such as the equipment being difficult to use (requiring complex work tasks or disinfection of the parts for every use) or being time-consuming [16].

The design of the ICU should prevent the distraction caused by the high level of noise in the ICU. It is also shown that noise may cause an increased stress level for the ICU staff [18, 38]. Moreover, it is also stated by the Occupational Health and Safety Administration that 20% of the workers may have a significant change in hearing if they are exposed to 90dBA noise for 8 h per day for 40 years [18].

Poor lighting in the ICU can cause discomfort while ICU workers are performing their daily tasks. Suitable lighting must consider the ideal level of lighting in different parts of the ICUs. Suitable lighting in the ICU varies as the lighting in the entrance and the waiting area is recommended to be 150 lx, circulation areas to be between 100 and 150 lx, and offices to be 750 lx. A direct interference with vision must be prevented and glare must be minimised. The nurse desks and monitoring areas should be located where light can be received in a 90° angle [12].

Heating and air conditioning in the ICUs are important physical conditions that affect the body temperature and cause heat stress in the ICU workers. Changes in the body temperature and heart rate along with sweating are known as the symptoms of the heat strain. This type of physiological strain indicates a cardiovascular response to the blood flow need. In the conditions where heat and ventilation in the ICU environment are not within ideal limits, the body starts to remove heat primarily by evaporation by sweating, the rate of which varies with air motion, humidity and type of clothing. The heat strain may primarily cause discomfort, but also induces heat-related disorders and acute musculoskeletal injuries [19]. The ideal temperature for workplaces is recommended as between 19° and 23°C but may vary in different settings [13].

Humidity is another factor in the working environment that affects workers' health. In conditions when humidity is low, it means the air is dry and can cause stuffy nose, dry and itchy skin, sore eyes, sore throat and flu-like symptoms in further cases. The relative humidity is stated as to be maintained between 40 and 70% [13].

3.2. Working conditions

Patients in ICUs receive continuous medical care 24 h a day from the ICU team. There are many different work tasks and related workload in the ICU setting. The influence of excessive workload in the ICU setting may result in a high level of stress, job dissatisfaction and physical injuries [20]. There is a direct correlation between the length of the shifts and the burnout due to excessive workload and fatigue. There are evidence and standards that consider the number of patients to be assigned to the ICU workforce. The evidence for the intensivist-to-patient ratios is ideally no higher than 1:14 inasmuch as it affects the staff well-being and patient care [21]. In a study investigating the clinical intensive care service, it was claimed that the paediatricians-to-patient ratio was 1:13, median working hours of the paediatricians were 60 h in a week, and indicated night shifts were 60 nights in a year [22]. The recommended nurse-to-patient rate is 1:1 for the critical patients with mechanical ventilation, and the maximum number of the patients to be assigned to a nurse is two according to the American College of Critical Care Medicine [23]. Those standards may vary with the national regulations in different countries. For example, the nurse-to-patient standard in Turkey is 1:4 for ICUs, not considering the dependency levels of the patients [5].

Studies in the literature show that there is a correlation between increased workload and increased medical errors and hospital infections [24]. Moreover, there is a relation between increased workload and death rates of the patients in the ICU. The excessive workload in the ICU setting is the main risk factor for hospital infections such as pneumonia, urinary tract infections, bloodstream infections, and surgical-site infections [25]. It is stated in the literature that when the ICU nurses give care to one patient above the recommended number, there is an increased risk for pulmonary failure by 53%, for nosocomial pneumonia by 7%, for unplanned extubation by 45% and for mortality rates by 9% [24]. In this context, the workload of the healthcare professionals in the ICU has crucial importance not only for causing occupational health problems, but also for patient safety issues [5, 24, 26].

The working characteristics in the ICU which require long work schedules lead to physical and mental fatigue [3]. Moreover, the long shifts (12 h and above) increase the errors and near misses, and decrease staff vigilance. As a further matter, the negative effects of shift work have been discussed for a long time, and are accepted as detrimental. It has a negative impact on individuals' health, such as disrupting the circadian rhythms, causing sleep disorders, causing increased risk of gastrointestinal tract disorders, increasing stress levels, altering activity and rest patterns and affecting the social and domestic life [27, 28]. Moreover, it disturbs the body's chemical and hormonal functions because of the fact that individuals working during the night are not able to benefit from the daylight. In many studies, it is discussed that working in night shifts for a long term increases the risk of breast cancer [29].

Nevertheless, the low salaries for healthcare professionals working in the ICU are not satisfying compared to the required working conditions [3].

2

3.3. Psychosocial factors

There are various psychosocial risk factors in ICU settings, such as high qualitative and quantitative demands, emotional demands, low job control, role conflicts, ambiguity, mobbing and physical violence, which affect ICU workers' well-being [30].

Intensive care units are stressful settings inasmuch as they require communicating with patients and their families facing the death and loss processes, coping with complex work tasks and adapting to busy work conditions [26]. The psychological hazards in the ICU may cause psychosocial burden, shifts in the mood, sadness, negative outlook towards life in general, irritation, loss of confidence and negative self-image [3]. Those negative conditions are related to symptoms of a high level of stress. Consequences of high levels of stress in the ICU can cause increased absence, lowered productivity, more accidents and physical injuries, higher job turnover and increased costs [30].

The ICU team members may encounter uncertainties, varied situations that require immediate action, high level of knowledge, psychomotor and cognitive skills and competences which may cause fatigue [3]. Lack of equipment and resources in the ICU may result in job dissatisfaction for the healthcare professionals working there [20]. In the studies done with anaesthesiologists and ICU nurses, it is found that overall nurses and the female anaesthesiologists consider the lack of resources as a cause for job dissatisfaction [2, 20].

Intensive care unit workers are responsible for many complex work processes in acute and chronic settings. There might be some role conflicts and ambiguity that result in decreased job control, misunderstanding and increased stress. However, in some cases, it is reported that physical aggression and physiological violence occur due to working in intense work conditions. Negative behaviours such as yelling, offending, ignoring, threatening or hiding important information can mean mobbing which are inadmissible for members of the ICU team. Being a victim of mobbing leads to physical and mental problems such as high level of stress, depression, eating disorders, addiction and suicide attempts [30].

The social hazards in the ICU setting are usually generated by working long shifts which require working at night and weekends. They may cause isolation from family relationships, social life difficulties, overall disinterest towards others, uncontrolled aggressiveness and difficulty in making decisions regarding personal life [3].

3.4. Ergonomic factors

Ergonomics are defined as the "laws of the work" and it primarily focuses on the physical aspects of the work. There are many force and energy requirements for work tasks in the ICU setting and there must be considerations of biomechanical rules and workplace adjustments to prevent ICU workers from musculoskeletal disorders [31].

Occupational musculoskeletal disorders not only occur in acute conditions but also may develop on account of cumulative micro traumas usually in relation to lack of *balance* of the body for tissue repair and adaptation to physical stress [32, 33].

Intensive care unit settings require physical loads on ICU workers during patient care [34, 35]. The physical hazards may cause ergonomic risks, which lead to musculoskeletal symptoms and disorders. Several conditions such as excessive and repetitive traumas while pushing and pulling heavy equipment, standing for long periods of time, not having adequate rest, manually lifting and moving partially or fully dependent patients in awkward, twisted or extremely bent positions requiring extreme muscular exertions must be considered as the major factors for musculoskeletal disorders [31, 34, 35]. The symptoms are mostly seen as pain in the leg, back, shoulder, neck and other parts of the body [3, 16].

In ICUs where the physical characteristics were not designed properly, healthcare professionals have a higher risk of musculoskeletal injuries due to repeated physical loads during patient care [34]. The ICU members with musculoskeletal symptoms are less productive because of pain and limited mobility, and they are likely to make consistent safety mistakes. Hence, they may also affect the health or endanger the safety of other members of ICU [31].

3.5. Biological factors

The ICU workers have increased risk related to biological hazards since they are exposed to infectious organisms during invasive and non-invasive procedures. Transmission of infectious agents can occur through blood and body fluids on equipment or their droplets' absorption by skin or mucosa through direct or indirect contact or lung penetration through the air. Intensive care unit work tasks and processes require direct or indirect contact with biological materials that results in illness and disease [13]. As in many other healthcare units, ICUs have the highest rate of needle stick injuries in the nursing workforce that can result in transmission of most common blood-borne infections such as Hepatitis B and C, other Hepatitis infections and HIV. Other infections can transmit to ICU workers by spreading through close contact and by droplets, such as tuberculosis and meningococcal meningitis [12, 36].

There are standard and transmission-based regulations in healthcare facilities to prevent infections occurring in the ICU workforce. Standard precautions include hand washing, respiratory hygiene and cough etiquette, waste management and decontamination, and appropriate use of personal protective equipment. Transmission-based interventions include airborne, contact and droplet precautions [13].

3.6. Chemical factors

The ICU workers face chemical hazards such as being exposed to antiseptic and disinfectants or inhaling their gases. During the work tasks and processes in the ICU settings, ICU workers can be exposed to surface cleaners, antiseptic solutions and anaesthetic gases such as formaldehyde. The exposure can occur through many routes, which commonly happens by penetration after lung inhalation, absorption by skin or mucosa contact through eyes or nose. They can cause inflammation or irritation on the part where contact occurred. Moreover, it can lead to dermatitis, allergic reactions (i.e. sneezing and rhinitis), asthma and cancer [13].

The effect of chemicals in the workplace can vary depending on some factors such as age, sex, ethnicity, genetics, immune system, nutrition, disease history, occupational history, previous exposures, other exposures to synergistic or antagonistic chemicals and recently used medications [12]. The occupational health and safety team in the hospital should keep records of all chemical agents which are being used in the ICU, and prepare emergency action plans in acute and chronic exposure cases.

4. Risks related to the ICU workers

4.1. Personal factors

There are some personal factors related to occupational diseases acquired by ICU workers. These factors can be summarised as ageing, inadequate physical condition, smoking and obesity.

The workforce in the ICU is ageing since the healthcare industry workforce is getting older in accordance with an increase in the retirement age requirements in all industries (around the world). In the United States, the average age of registered nurses is 46.8 [9]. The ageing workforce in the ICU might face increased risks for physical injuries and musculoskeletal disorders due to decreased muscular endurance and physical strength by age 50 and above [31]. Moreover, the workforce in the ICU is likely to have more chronic diseases with the ageing population [37].

The demographic characteristics of the society have changed in recent years. The body weight in certain populations is increasing rapidly. People's lifestyle is changing and it is leading to less healthy eating and having a more sedentary life. Obesity may cause many health problems such as back pain, osteoarthritis, diabetes mellitus, hyperlipidaemia, coronary heart diseases and other health conditions [37]. Considering the population trends, it has been shown that the body weight of ICU workers has also changed, and they are more likely to have obesity-related health problems and are at an increased risk of musculoskeletal injuries. Similarly, patients in the ICU have become heavier. Thus, this situation increases the risk of physical injuries of the ICU workforce while lifting or moving or transferring heavy patients [31].

4.2. Personal habits

The work tasks in the ICU setting require intense physical activity during the shift, even without lunch breaks or other breaks in some cases. Healthcare professionals who work in the ICU get fatigued after working for long hours. There are some personal habits that affect the level of physical or mental tiredness of the ICU workforce.

Studies have shown that regular physical activity prevents musculoskeletal disorders by maintaining flexibility of muscles and ligaments. According to this, ICU workers with a habit of regular physical activity have a decreased risk of physical injuries and musculoskeletal disorders [16, 38].

Intensive care unit workers might face sleeping disorders due to working night shifts. The high level of stress and physical tiredness after working for long hours might cause sleep disturbances in ICU workers [3]. Moreover, having inadequate sleep and rest increases the risk of unsafe practices and occupational accidents. It is shown in the studies that, there is a direct relation between sleep and level of attention [28].

Negative stress and poor balance between work and social life can cause careless dietary habits. A poor lifestyle implies a poor diet, which is not only related to eating too much or little, but also eating low-quality foods such as fast food and frozen food [13].

There is evidence about the correlation between an unhealthy lifestyle and decreased physical and mental abilities for work tasks [39]. Positive lifestyle such as having adequate sleep/rest, healthy eating habits and regular physical exercise affects job security and occupational quality [40].

4.3. Cognitive features

The cognitive features include individual differences, perceptions and decision making and human error. Individuals differ from each other by personality, reliability, perceptions and self-awareness. Moreover, some people are more likely to make errors [41]. It is shown in the literature that there is a correlation between cognitive failures and accidents [40].

The ICU setting has many different hazards, and the perceptions, decisions, and capabilities of the ICU workers are crucial to avoid the risks related to them. Decision making is an important factor that affects the level of risks and prevents accidents when an ICU worker makes the right decision at the right time. Individuals' competence is also important. Although some people are very capable of avoiding errors, their physical ability and willingness impact dealing with hazards [41]. However, cognitive features are directly related to occupational stressors so they can easily be changed [40].

There are some workplace interventions recommended to control and manage risks in the ICU setting, and most of these interventions are focused on behaviour change processes [16]. However, there are some individual factors affecting staff's behaviour change. Self-efficacy is the ability of individuals to accomplish tasks with barriers to change that they encounter during the process of behaviour change. It is related to the level of control of individuals over situations that affect their health [42].

In the conditions when the perceived self-efficacy level is high, the individual will realise the priority of the occupational health and safety principles to prevent work-related injuries or disorders while managing their work tasks [42].

There are some factors related to self-efficacy that affect the individual's behaviour change process negatively, such as decreased awareness of the benefits of the change and loss of interest or having a high level of perceived barriers to change (i.e. claiming to not have proper facilities for physical activity or complaining about time pressure while doing their work tasks) [42].

4.4. Occupational and health history

Risks arising from the previous workplace affect ICU workers' current health conditions. Some biological and chemical agents require a long period of time before causing any signs and symptoms while they are affecting the body functions. A detailed employment history provides information about the current occupational diseases and future health problems which might occur while performing in the ICU [10, 41].

Illnesses might have many causes such as ageing, lifestyle or genetic characteristics or viruses. Intensive care unit workers lose work days due to common illnesses i.e. symptoms of musculoskeletal disorders, headaches, dental issues, infectious diseases, gastric problems, among others. The health history of the ICU workers needs be recorded and comorbidities should be considered in relation to risk factors in the ICU [13].

5. Occupational health and safety practices in the ICU

The work tasks and processes in the ICUs are identified in a variety of guidelines prepared by the ILO (International Labour Organisation) and OSHA (Occupational Health and Safety Administration). The measures and practices related to protecting the ICU workers' health are identified in these guidelines. The measures and practices can be divided into two main topics such as workplace interventions and personal measures. Workplace interventions can be summarised as reducing the working hours and workload, designing and organising the work environment properly. Personal measures include staff training, providing risk management and health promotion programmes and other measures.

5.1. Workplace interventions

5.1.1. Reducing the working hours and workload

Changing work patterns and improving control strategies will result in decreased risks and reduced health deficits among ICU workers. Evidence shows that re-arranging working hours and workload results in reduced occupational health symptoms of the ICU workers. Improved working conditions, material and moral support, properly managed work shifts provide a safe environment in the ICU setting [40]. The occupational and safety team members have responsibilities to recognise workplace hazards and identify risks in the ICU setting that impact workplace practices and the workers' health status [10].

5.1.2. Designing and organising the work environment

A positive work environment is linked to improved patient and staff outcomes such as decreased hospital infections, death rates, and increased motivation and job satisfaction [43, 44].

The occupational health and safety team are involved in designing work equipment and ICU work process. Moreover, studies show that in situations where ICU workers' opinions were asked on the process of redesigning the unit, there was a significant increase in job satisfaction of staff and a dramatic reduction in turnover and absenteeism [10, 30].

5.1.3. Other interventions

Workplace interventions designed to prevent hazards and reduce related risks allow the occupational and safety team to implement strategies to improve safety culture in the ICU [44]. Safety culture is described as *"the product of individual and group values, attitudes, perceptions, competencies, and patterns of behaviour that determine the commitment of an organisation's health and safety management"* [45]. There is a direct connection between safety culture and trusted communication in the organisation. Moreover, increased perception of the importance of safe practices and sufficient confidence in preventive measures are remarked as the fundamentals of the safety culture [44]. Studies in this area show that perceptions of ICU safety are influenced by factors such as opinions of the management, working conditions, job satisfaction, team work climate, stress recognition, and safety climate [46]. Thus, workplace interventions to manage occupational risk factors should be focused on improving the safety culture of the ICU setting. After being established, the safety culture can be improved by initiating different intervention strategies [44]. The safety culture is known as a two-way system between the management's responsibilities and employees' commitment to their duties, which can only be established by key strategies: control, cooperation, communication and professional competence [13].

Designing safety checklists is another intervention that results in improved patient and workforce outcomes. A safety checklist aims to monitor safety performance and make improvements to work systems [38]. There are different aspects to creating safety criteria since they may be related to organisational, personal or professional characteristics. The safety hazards that threaten patient safety as well as health, well-being and safety of the ICU workforce must be stated on the checklists [38].

5.2. Personal measures

5.2.1. Staff training

Staff training interventions include prevention programmes related to physical, psychological, chemical, biological, ergonomic and other hazards in the ICU setting. In recent years, the importance of health promotion programmes is becoming more recognised as workplaces provide occupational health and safety (OHS) team members with access to a large group of people, who have good inter-communication and facilities to exchange information. Workplace health promotion activities enable OHS team members to participate in continuous assessment of the healthy lifestyle behaviours of ICU workers and to develop specific training interventions for them [10].

Occupational and safety practices should appreciate the biological, psychological, and social characteristics of individuals considering that interventions in the workplace will be integrated into adult life and health. The ability of the staff to participate in the training productively is an important factor that contributes to the effectiveness of the intervention. There are studies showing the benefits of on-work training programmes [16]. In this case, ICU professionals would not be requested to participate in staff training sessions when they need to rest after working long hours. Additionally, it is discussed in the literature that the on-work training sessions are more successful when they are model based or combined with multiple interventions [47–49].

Training should include different time periods such as orientation programmes when workers start working in the ICU (pre-employment examinations); periodical training; condition-based training where ICU workers need information about an unexpected or unusual situation (e.g. when they were caring for patients with an epidemic disease); return to work programmes for staff who have been absent after having a workplace accident or long-term leave from the ICU; and other programmes [10, 41].

5.2.2. Risk management

Risk management programmes comprise planning, applying and evaluating personal, physical and organisational interventions that aim to assess and decrease occupational risks to employees [50–52]. In recent years, many studies have been done with the aim of identifying high-risk tasks; creating and implementing solutions to reduce these risks in the workplace. There is legislation in many countries, for different work areas as well as ICUs to implement risk analysis and management programmes. Risk assessment involves the assessment of the severity and likelihood of harm which arises from identified hazards [11, 13]. Risk assessment can be made by using both qualitative and quantitative methods. However, in relation to legislations in many countries, a written risk assessment should be done including the risk control measures such as elimination of hazards, engineering controls, administrative controls and distribution of personal protective equipment [13]. Risk assessment and management interventions in the ICU should be performed as general and job-specific controls [31]. Therefore, safety hazards affecting the ICU workforce should be assessed individually, considering the work task–specific hazards that they might face. For example, in relation to biological risks, hazardous materials and wastes must be disposed safely. Continuous monitoring should be performed for persons who come into contact with biological materials by handling, manufacturing or storing them [13].

Work-related musculoskeletal disorders are one of the most common occupational health problems seen in ICU workers. The literature shows that evidence-based interventions used in ergonomic risk management programmes such as body mechanics training, ergonomic guidelines, exercise programmes, cognitive-behavioural interventions, social support programmes and workplace adjustments were found to be effective in terms of reducing the ergonomic risks to ICU workers [33, 47, 48, 50, 51, 53–57].

5.2.3. Health screening

Health screenings of ICU workers should be done regularly. A detailed history of previous employment and a comprehensive assessment of the current occupational diseases should be performed when the staff start working in the ICU setting (pre-employment examinations). Eventually, it should be followed by periodical screenings, condition-based screenings (e.g. when they were caring for patients with an epidemic disease) and return to work screenings for workers who had a workplace accident or a long-term leave from the ICU [10, 41].

5.2.4. Health promotion programmes

Occupational hazards and risk factors in the ICU are not only associated with the workplace setting, but are also related to personal habits such as smoking, not having a healthy diet or inadequate physical activity. Therefore, risks related to personal factors can only be managed by conducting health promotion programmes in their workplace. Health promotion programmes in the ICU are valuable interventions when they are used proactively, developed, and managed/monitored by experienced health professionals [9]. Health promotion activities (i.e. programmes aimed at diet management, weight control, physical activity or coping with stress) in the ICU should be developed considering the needs of ICU workers. For example, conditions related to high level of stress can be managed by improving coping skills. Those skills can be improved through stress management, problem solving, relaxation, and self-awareness trainings [13, 30]. However, a good health promotion intervention should be based on a model (i.e. Pender's Health Promotion Model; Prochaska's Trans-theoretic Model; Green's PRECEDE-PROCEED Model) [58]. According to these models, there are some factors such as past experiences, unsuccessful attempts to change, self-efficacy, social support, self-awareness and readiness to change that affect the positive results that may be achieved by workplace health promotion programmes [58–60].

5.2.5. Other measures

There are other monitoring and prevention programmes in relation to risks arising from hazards in the ICU setting. Different forms of prevention can be applied for varied risks as follows:

- Limitation of risk sources

- Limitation of ICU workers' reactions towards hazardous conditions

- Treatment of injuries and harm caused by hazards, including monitoring the long-term effects [30]

The aim of the preventative measures and interventions is to strengthen how ICU workers deal with physical, chemical, biological, psychosocial and ergonomic hazards. Another form of risk prevention is the optimisation of task content in connection with job rotation, job enlargement, job enrichment and creation of autonomous work groups (**Table 1**) [30].

Optimisation	Main focus/action
Job rotation	Move workers to different stations regularly
Job enlargement	Merge similar jobs into larger modules
Job enrichment	Group basic tasks and control elements together and assign workers to higher tasks
Creation of autonomous work groups	Create independent worker groups and give them the responsibilities of larger job fragments

Table 1. Optimisation of task content.

6. Conclusion

The ICU environment may cause a number of health risks in relation to occupational hazards. The workplace hazards include the physical environment of the ICU, working conditions, psychosocial factors, ergonomic factors, biological factors and chemical factors. The occurrence of occupational health problems in ICU workers not only leads to burnout and decreased job satisfaction, but also affects patient care and increases the cost of treatment. Workplace interventions and personal measures should be done in terms of reducing hazards and related risks in the ICU setting. Increased employee participation should be considered in all risk management, monitoring, and prevention programmes. The contribution of ICU workers in these programmes will improve the effectiveness of the interventions associated with reducing health risks in the ICU settings.

Author details

Melek Nihal Esin[1] and Duygu Sezgin[2*]

*Address all correspondence to: dusezgin@gmail.com

1 Public Health Nursing Department, Florence Nightingale Nursing Faculty, Istanbul University, Istanbul, Turkey

2 Department of Nursing & Midwifery, Education & Health Sciences Faculty, University of Limerick, Limerick, Ireland

References

[1] Durbin Jr CG. Team model: Advocating for the optimal method of care delivery in the intensive care unit. Critical Care Medicine. 2006 Mar 1;**34**(3):S12-S17

[2] Türkmen E, Sevinç S, İlhan M. Intensive care units in Turkish hospitals: Do they meet the minimum standards? Nursing in Critical Care. 2014 Jan 1;**21**:5

[3] Shimizu HE, Couto DT, Merchán-Hamann E, Branco AB. Occupational health hazards in ICU nursing staff. Nursing Research and Practice. 2011 Feb 7;**2010**:1-6.

[4] Hawker FH. Female specialists in intensive care medicine: Job satisfaction, challenges and work-life balance. Critical Care and Resuscitation. 2016 Jun;**18**(2):125

[5] Sevinç S, Türkmen E, İlhan M. The nursing workforce in critical care units in university and private hospitals in Turkey. Training. 2014 Apr 1;**15**:16

[6] Laschinger H. 14. Organisational and health effects of workplace empowerment in health care settings. The Innovation Imperative in Health Care Organisations: Critical Role of Human Resource Management in the Cost, Quality and Productivity Equation. 2012:**221**;221-222

[7] Ulrich BT, Lavandero R, Woods D, Early S. Critical care nurse work environments 2013: A status report. Critical Care Nurse. 2014 Aug 1;**34**(4):64-79

[8] Schmalenberg C, Kramer M. Essentials of a productive nurse work environment. Nursing Research. 2008 Jan 1;**57**(1):2-13

[9] Bhattacharya A, McGlothlin JD, editors. Occupational Ergonomics: Theory and Applications. Clark DR. Workstation Evaluation and Design. CRC Press; 2012 Mar 8. pp. 294, 302

[10] Sines D, Aldridge-Bent S, Fanning A, Farrelly P, Potter K, Wright J. Community and Public Health Nursing. John Wiley & Sons; 2013. pp. 192-193

[11] Health and safety essentials booklet. University of Limerick and NUI Galway, (nd) Ireland. p. 6

[12] Aw TC, Gardiner K, Harrington JM. Occupational Health (Pocket Consultant). 5th ed. USA: Blackwell Publishing; 2007. pp. 63-68, 73, 144

[13] Safety and Health at Work (QQI Level 5). Dublin: Nifast, Gill & McMillan; 2015. pp. 6-8, 54-58, 67-70, 77-78, 83-90

[14] Huisman ER, Morales E, Van Hoof J, Kort HS. Healing environment: A review of the impact of physical environmental factors on users. Building and Environment. 2012 Dec 31;**58**:70-80

[15] Koradecka, D, editor. Handbook of Occupational safety and health. In: Myrcha K, Gierasimiuk J, editors. Mechanical Hazards. USA: CRC Press; 2010. pp. 360-366

[16] Sezgin D, Esin MN. Predisposing factors for musculoskeletal symptoms in intensive care unit nurses. International Nursing Review. 2015 Mar 1;**62**(1):92-101

[17] Olausson S, Ekebergh M, Österberg SA. Nurses' lived experiences of intensive care unit bed spaces as a place of care: A phenomenological study. Nursing in Critical Care. 2014 May 1;**19**(3):126-134

[18] Bhattacharya A, McGlothlin JD, editors. Occupational ergonomics: Theory and applications. In: Grinshpun SA, Kim J, Murphy WJ, editors. Noise Exposure and Control. USA: CRC Press; 2012 Mar 8. pp. 792-793

[19] Bhattacharya A, McGlothlin JD, editors. Occupational ergonomics: Theory and applications. In: Bernard TE, editor. Occupational Heat Stress. USA: CRC Press; 2012 Mar 8. pp. 738-739

[20] Shidhaye RV, Divekar DS, Goel G, Shidhaye R. Influence of working conditions on job satisfaction in Indian anesthesiologists: A cross sectional survey. Anaesthesia Pain & Intensive Care. 2011 Jun 1;**15**(1):30-37

[21] Ward NS, Afessa B, Kleinpell R, Tisherman S, Ries M, Howell M, Halpern N, Kahn J, Members of Society of Critical Care Medicine Taskforce on ICU Staffing. Intensivist/patient ratios in closed ICUs: A statement from the Society of Critical Care Medicine Taskforce on ICU Staffing. Critical Care Medicine. 2013 Feb 1;**41**(2):638-645

[22] Radabaugh CL, Ruch-Ross HS, Riley CL, Stockwell JA, Conway Jr EE, Mink RB, Agus MS, Poss WB, Salerno RA, Vernon DD. Practice patterns in pediatric critical care medicine: Results of a workforce survey. Pediatric Critical Care Medicine. 2015 Oct 1;**16**(8):e308-e312

[23] Brilli RJ, Spevetz A, Branson RD, Campbell GM, Cohen H, Dasta JF, Harvey MA, Kelley MA, Kelly KM, Rudis MI, Andre AC. Critical care delivery in the intensive care unit: Defining clinical roles and the best practice model. Critical Care Medicine. 2001 Oct 1;**29**(10):2007-2019

[24] Kane RL, Shamliyan T, Mueller C, Duval S, Wilt TJ. Nurse staffing and quality of patient care. Evidence Report Technology Assessment (Full Report). 2007 Mar;**151**:1-15

[25] Daud-Gallotti RM, Costa SF, Guimarães T, Padilha KG, Inoue EN, Vasconcelos TN, Rodrigues FD, Barbosa EV, Figueiredo WB, Levin AS. Nursing workload as a risk factor for healthcare associated infections in ICU: A prospective study. PloS One. 2012 Dec 27;**7**(12):e52342

[26] Endacott R. Intensive Care Medicine. The continuing imperative to measure workload in ICU: Impact on patient safety and staff well-being. 2012; **38**(9):1415-1417

[27] Aveyard, D. How do 12-hour shifts affect ICU nurses? Kai Tiaki Nursing New Zealand. 2016 December;**22**(11):34-36.

[28] Koradecka D, editor. Handbook of occupational safety and health. In: Zuzewicz K, editor. Shift Work. USA: CRC Press; 2010. pp. 501-508

[29] Kamdar BB, Tergas AI, Mateen FJ, Bhayani NH, Oh J. Night-shift work and risk of breast cancer: A systematic review and meta-analysis. Breast Cancer Research and Treatment. 2013 Feb 1;**138**(1):291-301

[30] Koradecka D, editor. Handbook of occupational safety and health. In: Widerszal-Bazyl M, editor. Psychosocial Risk in the Workplace and its Reduction. USA; CRC Press: 2010. pp. 60-73, 77-80

[31] Bhattacharya A, McGlothlin JD, editors. Occupational ergonomics: Theory and applications. In: Longmate AR, editor. Ergonomic Control Measures in the Health Care Industry. USA: CRC Press; 2012 Mar 8. pp. 599, 601, 614-617, 623-624

[32] Dale AM, Jaegers L, Buchholz B, Welch L, Evanoff BA. Using process evaluation to determine effectiveness of participatory ergonomics training interventions in construction. Work. 2012 Jan 1;**41**(Supplement 1):3824-3826

[33] Côté JN, Ngomo S, Stock S, Messing K, Vézina N, Antle D, Delisle A, Bellemare M, Laberge M, St-Vincent M. Quebec research on work-related musculoskeletal disorders: Deeper understanding for better prevention. Industrial Relations/Relations Industrielles. 2013 Oct 1;**68**(4):643-660

[34] Freimann T, Merisalu E, Pääsuke M. Effects of a home-exercise therapy programme on cervical and lumbar range of motion among nurses with neck and lower back pain: A quasi-experimental study. BMC Sports Science, Medicine and Rehabilitation. 2015 Dec 4;**7**(1):31

[35] Ganiyu SO, Olabode JA, Stanley MM, Muhammad I. Patterns of occurrence of work-related musculoskeletal disorders and its correlation with ergonomic hazards among health care professionals. Nigerian Journal of Experimental and Clinical Biosciences. 2015 Jan 1;**3**(1):18

[36] Koradecka D, editor. Handbook of occupational safety and health. In: Dutkiewicz J, editor. Biological Agents. USA: CRC Press; 2010. pp. 386-388, 395-396

[37] Watkins D, Cousins J, editors. Public Health and Community Nursing: Frameworks for Practice. USA: Elsevier Health Sciences; 2009 Oct 23

[38] Bowie P, Ferguson J, MacLeod M, Kennedy S, de Wet C, McNab D, Kelly M, McKay J, Atkinson S. Participatory design of a preliminary safety checklist for general practice. British Journal of General Practice. 2015 May 1;**65**(634):e330-e343

[39] El Fassi M, Bocquet V, Majery N, Lair ML, Couffignal S, Mairiaux P. Work ability assessment in a worker population: Comparison and determinants of Work Ability Index and Work Ability score. BMC Public Health. 2013 Apr **8**;13(1):305

[40] Abbasi M, Zakerian A, Kolahdouzi M, Mehri A, Akbarzadeh A, Ebrahimi MH. Relationship between Work Ability Index and cognitive failure among nurses. Electronic Physician. 2016 Mar;**8**(3):2136

[41] Boyle T. Health and Safety: Risk Management. USA: Routledge; 2015 Sep 14.

[42] Larsson A, Karlqvist L, Westerberg M, Gard G. Identifying work ability promoting factors for home care aides and assistant nurses. BMC Musculoskeletal Disorders. 2012 Jan 11;**13**(1):1

[43] Vigorito MC, McNicoll L, Adams L, Sexton B. Improving safety culture results in Rhode Island ICUs: Lessons learned from the development of action-oriented plans. The Joint Commission Journal on Quality and Patient Safety. 2011;**37**(11):509-514

[44] Chaboyer W, Chamberlain D, Hewson-Conroy K, Grealy B, Elderkin T, Brittin M, McCutcheon C, Longbottom P, Thalib L. CNE article: Safety culture in Australian intensive care units: Establishing a baseline for quality improvement. American Journal of Critical Care. 2013 Mar 1;**22**(2):93-102

[45] Sorra JS, Nieva VF. Hospital Survey on Patient Safety Culture. Rockville, MD: Agency for Healthcare Research and Quality; September 2004. Prepared by Westat, under Contract 290-96-0004. AHRQ Publication 04-0041

[46] Sexton JB, Berenholtz SM, Goeschel CA, Watson SR, Holzmueller CG, Thompson DA, Hyzy RC, Marsteller JA, Schumacher K, Pronovost PJ. Assessing and improving safety climate in a large cohort of intensive care units. Critical Care Medicine. 2011 May 1;**39**(5):934-939

[47] Stigmar KG, Petersson IF, Jöud A, Grahn BE. Promoting work ability in a structured national rehabilitation program in patients with musculoskeletal disorders: outcomes and predictors in a prospective cohort study. BMC Musculoskeletal Disorders. 2013;**14**(1):1

[48] Rasmussen CD, Holtermann A, Mortensen OS, Søgaard K, Jørgensen MB. Prevention of low back pain and its consequences among nurses' aides in elderly care: A stepped-wedge multi-faceted cluster-randomized controlled trial. BMC Public Health. 2013;13(1):1088

[49] Lim HJ, Black TR, Shah SM, Sarker S, Metcalfe J. Evaluating repeated patient handling injuries following the implementation of a multi-factor ergonomic intervention program among health care workers. Journal of Safety Research. 2011;42(3):185-191

[50] Black TR, Shah SM, Busch AJ, Metcalfe J, Lim HJ. Effect of transfer, lifting, and repositioning (TLR) injury prevention program on musculoskeletal injury among direct care workers. Journal of Occupational and Environmental Hygiene. 2011 Jan 22;8(4):226-235

[51] Rivilis I, Van Eerd D, Cullen K, Cole DC, Irvin E, Tyson J, Mahood Q. Effectiveness of participatory ergonomic interventions on health outcomes: A systematic review. Applied Ergonomics. 2008 May 31;39(3):342-358

[52] Yildiz AN, Çaman ÖG, Nihal ES. İşyerinde sağliği geliştirme programlari. Ankara: TÜRK-İŞ; 2012

[53] Silverstein B, Clark R. Interventions to reduce work-related musculoskeletal disorders. Journal of Electromyography and Kinesiology. 2004 Feb 29;14(1):135-152

[54] Sato N, Sekiguchi M, Kikuchi S, Shishido H, Sato K, Konno S. Effects of long-term corset wearing on chronic low back pain. Fukushima Journal of Medical Science. 2012;58(1):60-65

[55] Bigos SJ, Holland J, Holland C, Webster JS, Battie M, Malmgren JA. High-quality controlled trials on preventing episodes of back problems: Systematic literature review in working-age adults. The Spine Journal. 2009 Feb 28;9(2):147-168

[56] Roelofs PD, Bierma-Zeinstra SM, van Poppel MN, van Mechelen W, Koes BW, van Tulder MW. Cost-effectiveness of lumbar supports for home care workers with recurrent low back pain: An economic evaluation alongside a randomized-controlled trial. Spine. 2010 Dec 15;35(26):E1619–E1626

[57] Calmels P, Queneau P, Hamonet C, Le Pen C, Maurel F, Lerouvreur C, Thoumie P. Effectiveness of a lumbar belt in subacute low back pain: An open, multicentric, and randomized clinical study. Spine. 2009 Feb 1;34(3):215-220

[58] Pender NJ, Murdaugh CL, Parsons MA. Health Promotion in Nursing Practice. USA: 6th ed. 2006.

[59] Gielen AC, McDonald EM, Gary TL, Bone LR. Using the precede-proceed model to apply health behavior theories. Health Behavior and Health Education: Theory, Research, and Practice. 2008;4:407-429

[60] Prochaska JO, Velicer WF. The transtheoretical model of health behavior change. American Journal of Health Promotion. 1997 Sep;12(1):38-48

7

Videolaryngoscopy in the Intensive Care Unit: We could Improve ICU Patients Safety

Eugenio Martínez Hurtado,
Miriam Sánchez Merchante, Sonia Martín Ventura,
María Luisa Mariscal Flores and
Javier Ripollés Melchor

Abstract

Tracheal intubation is one of the most common and dangerous procedures in the intensive care units (ICU), and is usually done in more difficult conditions than in the operating room. Intubation failure can occur unexpectedly, and is the second most common event reflected in the ICU in the NAP4. Complications associated with airways were more likely to occur in ICU than in the operating room (severe hypoxemia, arrhythmia, hypotension, cardio-vascular collapse, etc.), and generates more frequent damage to the patient. The theoretical benefits of videolaryngoscopes, as proper and correct use, offer the potential to reduce the difficulty of intubation in the ICU. In recent years, the role of videolaryngoscopes in ICU has been the subject of debate. Numerous studies have shown increased morbidity when performing multiple attempts at tracheal intubation. Videolaryngoscopes allow a view of the entrance of glottis independent of the line of sight, and have also been shown to improve glottis and intubation success rates in emergency and emergency services, in the prehospital setting, and specifically in patients with known predictors of difficult airway (DA).

Keywords: tracheal intubation, NAP4, complications, videolaryngoscopes, difficult airway, airway management, laryngoscopy, critical patient

1. Introduction

Airway management (AM) in intensive care units (ICU) is a common practice that is usually performed in more complicated conditions than in the operating room, where it is performed on a scheduled basis. The fundamental difference is that these patients are frequently in a situation of

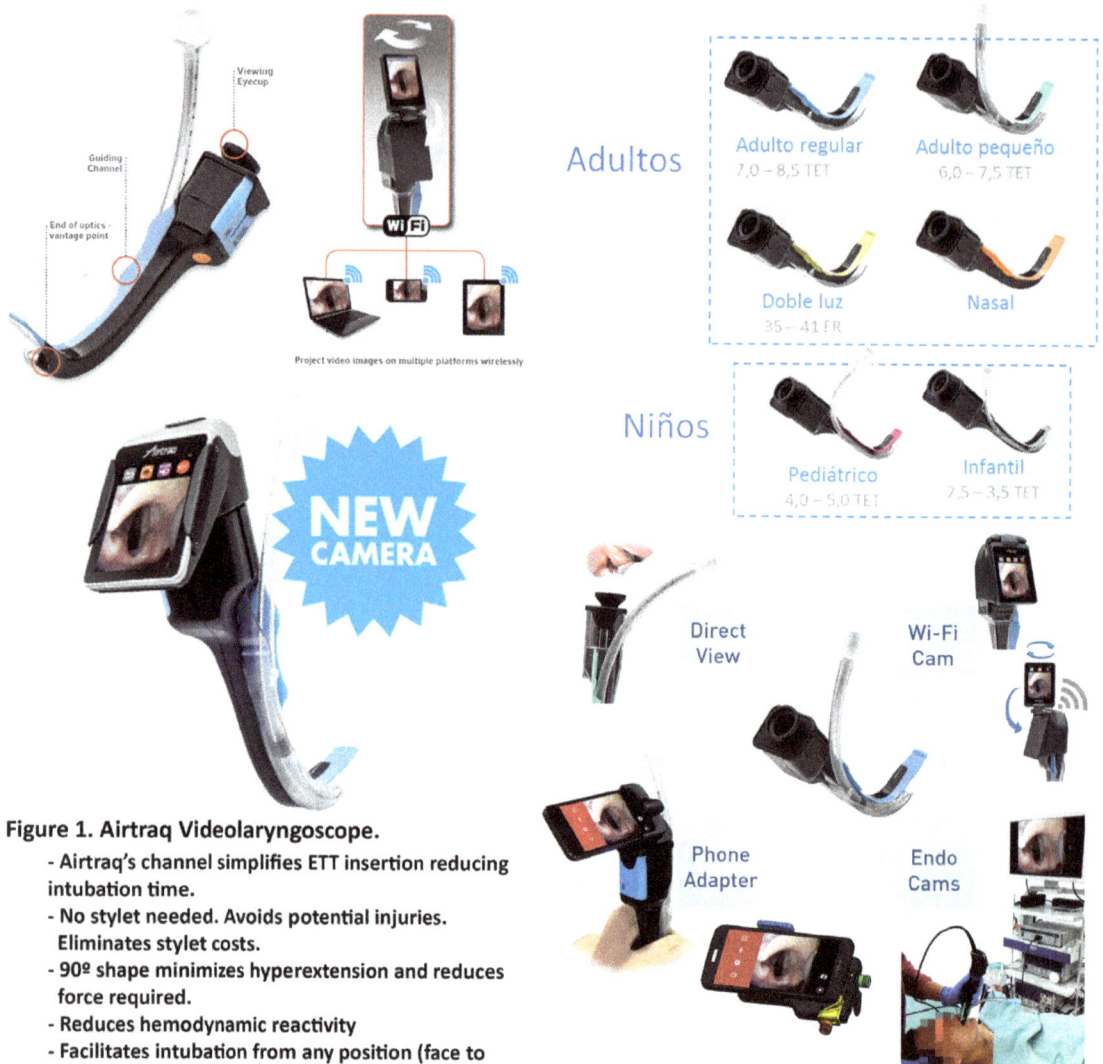

Figure 1. Airtraq Videolaryngoscope.
- Airtraq's channel simplifies ETT insertion reducing intubation time.
- No stylet needed. Avoids potential injuries. Eliminates stylet costs.
- 90º shape minimizes hyperextension and reduces force required.
- Reduces hemodynamic reactivity
- Facilitates intubation from any position (face to face, etc.).
- High intubation success rate in Difficult Airways.

Figure 1. Airtraq videolaryngoscope.

hypoxemia and cardiovascular collapse, so in many situations, the airway management in these clinical conditions is often complicated, if not emergency. Therefore, it is usually considered that these patients present, at the beginning, a possible difficult airway (DA).

Although failure to manage AM sometimes occurs unexpectedly, it is known to be the second most common event reflected in NAP4 in the ICU [1]. So, all patients admitted in the ICU should be considered at risk.

The airway approach in this environment has gained interest in recent years, especially after NAP4, in which airway complications were found to be more likely to occur in the ICU than in the operating room (severe hypoxemia, in addition to arrhythmias, hypotension, and cardiovascular collapse), and more frequently caused harm to the patient. This study specifically mentioned the theoretical benefit of videolaryngoscopes (VL), since their proper and correct use would offer the potential to reduce the difficulty of intubation in the ICU (**Figure 1**).

Other important conclusions drawn from the NAP4 were the scarce airway assessment performed in the critical units and did not allow us to anticipate a DA, resulting in poor planning. It was also observed that, in the context of an unexpected DA, the limited ability to modify the established plan may lead to a failure to resolve the situation.

The utility of videolaryngoscopy in anesthesia is widely recognized and endorsements advocating its use have been incorporated in the UK and American Difficult Airway Society guidelines [2, 3].

2. Epidemiology

The degree of difficulty with face mask ventilation (FMV) and intubation with direct laryngoscopy (DL) is very variable according to the studies and although the degree of difficulty for intubation does not have to correspond to the difficulty for ventilation with facial masks, if they occur together in the same patient, the consequences can be catastrophic [4].

Traditionally, the difficulty for laryngoscopy vision is difficult to intubate [5, 6].

In general, the incidence of Cormack-Lehane grades 3/4 and 4/4 ranges from 1 to 10%, and 2–8%, respectively. These figures are up to 7.9% in pregnant women requiring general anesthesia, with 2% of cases being *"very difficult intubation"*, an incidence similar to difficult orotracheal intubation (OTI) in urgent non-obstetric surgical patients.

Finally, the catastrophic situation of *"can't-intubate-can't-oxygenate"* (CICO) can occur with an incidence of 1–3 per 10,000 patients to 1 per 50,000 patients according to the authors.

All these figures vary between studies, mainly because there is no unanimity in the definitions or terms related to AM.

Within the specific context of an ICU, the incidence of DA rises to 10–20% [7–12].

Facial mask ventilation (FMV) is a fundamental element of the AM that would ensure patient oxygenation between the different intubation attempts. It has been classically described an incidence of difficulty FMV of 0.08% [5].

In 2004, a scale of 4 degrees of difficulty FMV was established, assigning a score of 0–4 according to the difficulty found [13], which was later used in a study of 22,660 patients [14], Finding a degree of difficulty of:

- Grade 1: easy FMV (77.4%).

- Grade 2: easy FMV with an oral cannula or other adjuvants (21.1%).

- Grade 3: difficult FMV (inadequate, unstable or requiring two operators) (1.4%).

- Grade 4: inability FMV (0.16%).

- Grade 3 or 4 + difficult intubation: 0.37%.

In order to increase statistical power in some variables of the previous study, in 2009, a new study was carried out, collecting more than 50,000 patients [15]. It was recognized that the incidence of impossible FMV, defined as *"the inability to ventilate with facial masks despite the use of facilitating devices and 2-hand ventilation"*, was found to be around 0.15%.

3. Particularities of airway management in the critical patient

Critical patient intubation is often performed in ICU, but can also be performed in locations away from the operating room, where working conditions and available materials are often inadequate. The difficulty rate of orotracheal intubation in emergency situations is 3 times higher than the programmed procedure, with a reported incidence of 10–20% failure at the first-attempt [7], with a complication rate 50 times higher than those found during anesthesia [1].

The AM of the critically ill patient may be complicated by the anatomical characteristics involving the visualization of glottis opening, or the difficult passage of the tracheal tube through the vocal cords, or by the clinical situation itself, which may contribute to the cardio-vascular collapse. Among these causes of physiologic DA are hypoxemia, hypotension, severe metabolic acidosis, and right ventricular failure [16]. In fact, approximately 20% of patients in the ICU will experience critical hypoxemia, which, in the worst case, leads to death. Other common complications are esophageal intubation, aspiration, and selective bronchial intubation, among others.

DA is defined as *"that clinical situation in which an experienced anesthesiologist present difficulties with ventilation with a face mask, difficulty with OTI, or both"*. Likewise, difficult intubation can be defined as *"the need for 3 or more attempts for OTI, or more than 10 minutes to achieve it"* [2].

However, despite handling the DA forced to take decisions and perform actions quickly and effectively, the truth is that there is no unanimity in the definitions or terms related to AM, because "the DA not exists, in reality, but is a complex interaction between the patient, the anesthetist, the available equipment and other circumstances" [17].

Until a few years ago, the available systems of evaluation have had in little consideration factors not related to the patient. Some factors that complicate and diminish the safety of the management of the AM such as:

- Experience.

- Pressure of time-urgency.

- Availability of suitable equipment.

- Location.

- Human factors.

However, it is currently considered *"management of context-sensitive airway"*, where a gaseous exchange is more valued than the tracheal intubation itself [18], which consists of four ventilation and oxygenation methods:

1. Facial mask.

2. Supraglottic or extraglottic devices.

3. Endotracheal tube.

4. Surgical AM.

The use of any of these methods depends not only on the devices but also on the situation facing the professional. In this management of context-sensitive MA, maintenance of the patient's gauche exchange is the priority and should not be *"device dependent"*. Thus, careful evaluation of the *"context"* interpretation is essential for the safe practice of MA management.

The concept *"context-sensitive AM"* acquires special relevance in critically ill patients, and there are several causes that make it difficult to manage their AM:

1. Non-patient dependent:

   - Who manages airway?

   - Where is the patient?

   - What equipment and medication are available?

   - Who helps?

2. Dependent patient:

   - Predictive tests of AD.

   - Pathology of the patient (hemorrhage, edema, trauma, increased secretions, etc.).

4. Complications of intubation in the critical patient

The primary indication for OTI in ICU is the acute respiratory failure. Weakness and fatigue of respiratory muscles (ventilatory failure) and disruption of gas exchange (respiratory failure) are common, and the risk of hypoxemia and cardiovascular shock during the OTI process is high, ranging from 15 to 50%.

Critical patient intubation presents life-threatening complications in more than one-third of cases [19]. The most common are respiratory and hemodynamic alterations [20]. The main adverse event associated with the technique is hypoxemia with a dramatic decrease in peripheral oxygen saturation (SapO2) despite adequate preoxygenation. In almost half of the cases, the indication for tracheal intubation is due to an acute respiratory failure with a previous SapO2 of less than 90% that supports the appearance of severe hypoxemia.

The second complication due to its frequency is hemodynamic alteration with hypotension after intubation, associated or not with desaturation. Mort reported 60 cardiac arrests during 3035 intubations outside the operating room (incidence of 2%) [21]. About 83% of these patients experienced severe hypoxemia (SatpO2 < 70%). The choice of the drug suitable for anesthetic induction is very important to minimize hypotension in the critical.

Other complications described in the literature are esophageal intubation and pulmonary aspiration. The former increases the risk of cardiac arrest by 15 times.

NAP4 reported that ICU, far from representing a safe place to operate the airway, were a place of potential danger. Airway-related complications were more likely to occur in the ICU than in the operating room, and more often resulted in harm to the patient. Thus, the rate of airway complications that appeared in the ICU was more than 50 times higher than those found during anesthesia, and 61% of the ICU patients reported on NAP4 suffered neurological damage or death, compared to 14% during the anesthetic procedure and 33% in the emergency department. Although most of the potentially fatal airway events in the ICU were due to especially tracheal tube displacement or tracheostomy (especially in obese patients), difficulties were also identified associated with esophageal intubation, rapid sequence intubation, and failure techniques of the rescue of the airways [1].

There are four factors that are independently associated with a serious complication during the procedure:

1. Age is a factor that cannot be modified and is accompanied by a worse response of the organism to any aggression.

2. Second, there are two factors depending on the patient's previous physiological status, the presence of hypotension, and/or hypoxemia conditions an increased risk of complications. In some cases, these factors can be modified by optimizing blood pressure and oxygenation.

3. The presence of secretions in the oropharyngeal cavity hinders laryngoscopic vision and has been associated with an increase in the rate of failure of tracheal intubation.

4. Lastly, the need for more than one attempt for intubation increases the risk of complications. A number greater than two attempts increases the risk of hypoxemia, bradycardia, aspiration of gastric contents, and cardiac arrest exponentially [21].

The presence of two clinicians reduces the risk of complications.

5. Approach of the airway management in the critical patient

The aims of the AM, understood as the accomplishment of maneuvers and the use of devices that allow adequate and safe ventilation to patients who need it, is to guarantee the oxygenation in a situation of potential vital risk for that patient.

The optimal AM and ventilation of critical patients remain a basic pillar in survival, evolution, and prognosis, with OTI being the gold standard in these situations.

Most patients requiring tracheal intubation and mechanical ventilation in the ICU are, in contrast to those requiring these procedures in an operating room, patients with a circulatory and/or respiratory compromise. Therefore, the intubation procedure should be non-aggressive and atraumatic.

The cardiorespiratory instability usually presented by the seriously ill patient (with reduced functional residual capacity and safe apnea time), together with the urgent nature of the situation, the low predictability of the possible scenarios, jointly with the fact that it is often not possible ensure adequate gastric emptying, determine that the intubation of critical airway is a high-risk procedure. For this reason, all critical patients should be initially managed as potential AD.

The results of the NAP4 audit are parallel to other studies that consider that multiple attempts at intubation in the critical patient result in a high incidence of adverse events [22]. In order to limit the number of attempts to two and to ensure success, interventions such as an adequate patient position and the existence, at the bedside, of correct material equipment and experienced personnel are necessary.

The assessment of the airway in the critical patient may be complex, but adequate planning should be part of the daily approach to the airway. This assessment must include the factors that predict a DA that we routinely use in the anesthesia consultation. The patient's position, the additional help present, and the available material must be evaluated prior to anesthetic induction. In addition, the physiological characteristics of the subject such as the full stomach and situations that favor desaturation (obesity and pulmonary shunt) should be considered.

The oxygenation of patients before and during intubation is of paramount importance [23]. Premaneuver denitrogenate has been shown to be useful as oxygenation with nasal goggles during apnea. The administration of high concentrations of oxygen through high-flow nasal glasses (HFNG) seems to offer advantages over the classic preoxygenation models. It provides some degree of positive pressure even during laryngoscopy without requiring patient collaboration [24].

Historically, direct laryngoscopy has been the most commonly used method for intubation in critically ill patients. Alternatives such as luminous stylet, supraglottic device, and flexible fibrobronchoscope are hardly used outside the surgical area. VLs have been proposed as an initial approach by some authors, but their implementation is being limited and reserved as a rescue technique. It is true that these devices improve the vision of the glottis, but in less-experienced hands, they slow the procedure and, in critical patients with few reserves, additional few seconds can have fatal consequences.

6. Videolaryngoscopes in the ICU

In conventional airway management, routine OTI with traditional direct laryngoscopy (DL) is still the common practice [25, 26], with the Macintosh as standard gold DL, a device created just 10 years before the first ICU was Inaugurated by the anesthesiologist Bjorn Ibsen in Copenhagen (December 1953) [27, 28]. On the other hand, in DA cases, the technique of choice for intubation is the use of the fiber optic bronchoscopy (FOB), although there are more and more studies in which videolaryngoscopy is used as an alternative approach in induced/sleep or awake patient, since FOB is an expensive, fragile, and requires regular maintenance, is complex to dispose of in emergency situations or in prehospital emergencies, and requires previous training.

Failure of endotracheal intubation using Classical Direct Laryngoscopy with a Macintosh laryngoscope or other technique may occur unexpectedly. And, since the second most common event reflected in the NAP4 reports on the ICU was failed intubation, proper and correct use of videolaryngoscopes (VL) would offer the potential to reduce the difficulty of intubation in general in the ICU [1, 29].

Numerous studies have shown increased morbidity when performing multiple attempts at tracheal intubation. Videolaryngoscopes allow a view of the entrance of glottis independent of the line of sight (LI), especially those that have angled blades. The fact that the image sensor is in the distal part of the blade causes us to have a panoramic view of the glottis, without the need to *"align the axes"*, thus avoiding hyperextension of the head, and in practice having a Laryngoscopy Cormack-Lehane (CL) grade 1 or 2 (CL 1/4 or 2/4) in 99% of the cases (**Figure 2**).

VL have also been shown to improve glottis and intubation success rates in emergency and emergency services, in the prehospital setting, and specifically in patients with known predictors of DA [30].

However, achieving CL grade 1 laryngoscopy (CL 1/4) in laryngoscopy with a VL does not guarantee the success of OTI, which is relatively frequent in VLs that have a curved leaf, especially during the learning stage [31, 32].

Previous studies with novice and experienced anesthetists have suggested that the learning curve with an optical device can be around 20 applications to be competent to manage [33].

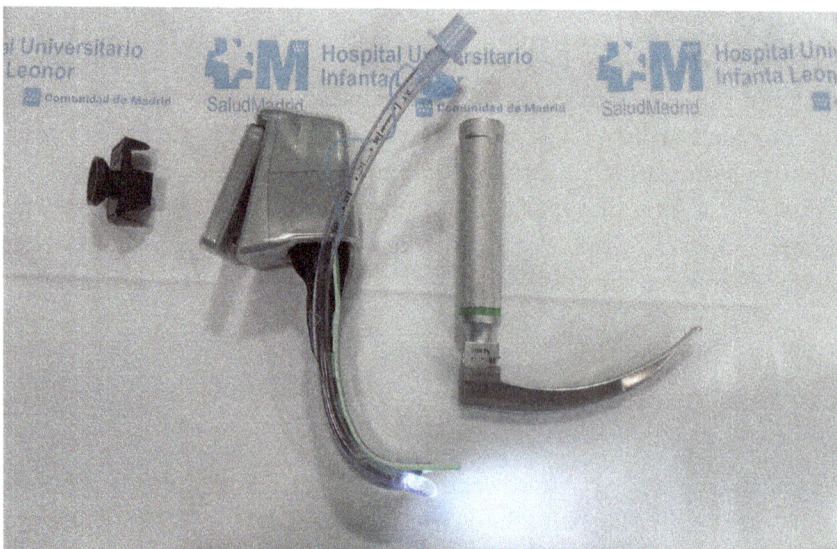

Figure 2. Glottic view differences.

Although these numbers are lower than those suggested by Greaves (80% of competence acquired with 30 cases, and complete with 100 cases), the video imaging technology of these new devices offers a shared vision between instructor and student [34], which can facilitate the teaching of airway anatomy, critical assessment of technique, and feedback. This may lead to skill acquisition faster than that achieved with traditional training with direct laryngoscopy [35].

This difficulty in achieving intubation despite the correct exposure of the larynx even in expert hands may be finally impossible, and success depends more on the operator's ability and patient's airway characteristics than on the own device [36]. However, in an attempt to overcome this problem, channeled videolaryngoscopes have the advantage of orienting the endotracheal tube (ETT) toward the trachea, allowing directed intubation with a little manipulation of the airway.

On the other hand, the evidence suggests that the use of indirect laryngoscopy (IL) improves the overall success rate of emergency/emergency tracheal intubation, as well as reduces the incidence of esophageal intubation when compared to conventional direct laryngoscopy (LD) [36].

In addition to this, we must mention that the VL, thanks to its good image quality, allow to easily recognize the structures of the larynx to achieve an image with a field between 45° and 60°, as opposed to the distant and tubular vision of the classical laryngoscopy (about 15°).

This image also allows to be certain about both the success of the intubation and the depth of insertion of the ETT, and can also easily recognize and correct esophageal intubation, a serious cause of morbidity and mortality. And another added advantage is that they provide an LED light, of greater luminous intensity than the conventional one and with a spectral irradiation closer to the human eye.

The NAP4 (the 4th National Audit Project on Major Complications in Airway Management in the UK) specifically mentions the theoretical benefit of videolaryngoscopes [1], with evidence that they can be more efficient than a Macintosh laryngoscope conventional.

For these and other reasons, these optical devices were incorporated into the airway management guidelines by the ASA as valid options in both the DA as usual, including, without excluding or limiting, laryngoscopes with different sizes and types of blades, VL, facial masks or supraglottic airway devices (SAD) such as laryngeal mask (LMA) or Fastrach® (ILMA), laryngeal tube, etc., fibrobronchoscope (FBO), extraglottic device (Frova, Eischman, etc.), nasal intubation, etc. [2].

6.1. Features

The characteristics that would define an ideal intubation device are described in **Table 1**.

During the last few years, many types of rigid, semi-rigid, optical, fiber optic and video-assisted laryngoscopes have been developed, as well as stiff and flexible stylets, as well as the classic flexible fibrobronchoscope, all of them with a common goal: to solve a classic problem for anesthesiologists, the difficult airway. The clinical evidences tell us about the real usefulness of all these devices in the solution of the problem for which they were designed. Scientific evidence of its use, the advantage of one over another, and the choice of each of them in a particular patient are yet to be determined.

- Light and portable.
- Economic and one-time use. Disposable, no risk of cross contamination.
- Short learning curve. Easy intubation with minimal skills.
- Good glottal visibility.
- Presence of an anti-fogging system that ensures the visualization of the airway despite the presence of secretions.
- Rapid orotracheal intubation, with minimal manipulation of the patient.
- Suitable for all types of ETT.
- Allow the administration of O_2/ventilate.
- Allow aspiration.
- It does not produce hemodynamic changes.
- Adaptable to the anatomy.
- Can be used with little mouth opening.
- Do not need cervical hyperextension.
- It can be used with the patient in any position.
- Possibility of connection to monitor for teaching.
- It can be used in awake patients.
- Multiple display options.
- Storage capacity and image integration.

Table 1. Characteristics of an ideal intubation device.

At the moment, all the VL present as common characteristics [37–44]:

1. *Technically*: they present a wider image, high resolution, with improvement of the degree of laryngoscopy. Indirect vision of the glottis can be obtained in different ways:

   (a) Camcorder whose digital image is transmitted to a screen of an external monitor.

   (b) Beam of optical fibers.

   (c) System of prisms, which transmit the image through a system of lenses.

2. *Procedure*: similar to the Macintosh or Miller laryngoscope, although on other occasions it is inserted through the midline, or fiber optic bronchoscope (FOB).

3. *Teaching*: allow to teach and show multiple visions, the assistant visualizes and can see the result of laryngeal manipulation. The procedure can be saved and remembered. It facilitates the learning of alternative techniques to FBO, etc.

4. *Research*: images can be stored.

5. *Comfort for the user*: more comfortable posture, less contact with secretions, blood, etc.

6.2. Classification

Resulting the classifications proposed by Pott et al. [43], Healy et al. [38], and Niforopoulou et al. [44], although all VLs allow a view of the entrance of glottis independent of the line of sight (indirect laryngoscopy [LI]), could be classified according to the type of blade [42]:

1. VL with *"Standard"* rigid blade, similar to the LD Macintosh such as the C-MAC (Karl Storz, Tuttligen, Germany) or McGrath MAC (Aircraft Medical, Edinburgh, UK), among others. Also used as a conventional direct laryngoscope. This reduces, at least theoretically, the learning curve needed to use them correctly.

Other advantages common to all of them are the ease of visualization of the glottic structures, which allow to use any type of endotracheal tube (ETT) and the longer duration than the fiberscope, combined with the lowest cost.

The disadvantage is that, even in most of cases CL improves, the introduction of ETT is sometimes difficult and a certain practice is required, so eventually ETT must be performed with a guarantor (contrary to which occurs with angled blades).

2. VL with *Angled Rigid Blade* such as Glidescope (Verathon, Bothell, WA, USA), king vision with no channel blades (KingSystems, www.Kingsystems.com, distributed in Spain by Ambu a/S, www.ambu.es), the McGrath MAC X blade (aircraft medical, Edinburgh, UK), or the C-MAC D blade (Karl Storz, Tuttligen, Germany), among others.

All of them present advantages common to all of them: ease of visualization of glottic structures, allow to use any type of ETT and longer duration than the fiberscope.

The disadvantage is that, although Cormack-Lehane improves in most cases, the introduction of ETT is sometimes difficult.

The lack of a channel in which to put the ETT usually requires a certain practice and, often, it is necessary to preform the ETT with a catcher that provides the same the angulation that has the blade of the VL so as to be able to direct it to the entrance of the glottis.

3. Videolaryngoscopes with *Channel to guide* the ETT such as Airtraq (Prodol Meditec, Vizcaya, Spain, 2005. US Patent No 6,843,769), King Vision with a channeled blade (KingSystems), and the Pentax-AWS-S100 (Pentax Corporation, Tokyo, Japan), among others.

They all have a channel through which the ETT slides for intubation. As the ETT is directed by the channel, we must do any modification of movements on the device and not on the tube.

The tube does not need to be preformed with a stylet and generally enhances the Cormack-Lehane.

6.3. Current scientific evidence

The new optical devices are recommended to improve the management of the airway, both in anesthetic care and in critical patients [41, 42, 45, 46]. In recent years, the role of videolaryngoscopes has been debated, especially its use in the ICU [29, 31, 37, 42, 47–51], where there is a lack of scientific evidence and, in general, intubation is performed in more complicated conditions than in the operating room [52]. However, this evidence is supported in the surgical setting as there are randomized controlled trials (RCTs), meta-analyses, and systematic reviews. Although the environments are different, neither the techniques for the acquisition of competencies, and in one place as in the other, there are situations of unexpected vital commitment and/or deterioration of respiratory and hemodynamic function [7, 21, 41, 53, 54]. Therefore, the results of existing studies in surgical areas can be extrapolated to the field of ICU for many of the above-mentioned plots.

In this sense, Healy et al. published an updated systematic review of Videolaringoscopes in 2012 with the objective of organizing the literature about the effectiveness of modern VL in the OTI and then performing a quality assessment and making recommendations for its use [38].

The comparison of VL with LD was based on three main results: global success, first-attempt success, and successful intubation time.

The vision of the glottis was a desirable result, but since with the VL the intubation can be performed despite having a limited view of it and, on the other hand, a good view of the larynx does not always guarantee a successful intubation, it was not considered a target for the recommendation.

The final recommendations of the study could be summarized in three points:

1. In patients at risk of difficult laryngoscopy, the use of Airtraq, C-Trach, GlideScope, Pentax AWS, and V-MAC is recommended for successful intubation.

2. The use of the Airtraq, Bonfils, Bullard, C-Trach, GlideScope, and Pentax AWS by an operator with reasonable prior experience is recommended for successful intubation in CLD (CL ≥ 3).

3. There is additional evidence to support the use of Airtraq, Bonfils, C-Trach, GlideScope, McGrath, and Pentax AWS after intubation failed by direct laryngoscopy to achieve successful intubation.

Be that as it may, the use of VLs not only improves glottic vision, and in the ICU they also present other advantages such as positive effects on teamwork, communication and knowledge of the situation, as well as on technical skills. The use of VL on the training of residents, with an adjunct that shares their opinion as responsible for intubation seen on the screen, giving advice to help intubation, training nurses of the ICU allowing them to control the effect of the pressure on the cricoid during the sellick, adjusting it as necessary. In addition, the VL is immediately available, which means an improvement in the management of the unexpected DA [37, 55].

A major advantage of standard "rigid" VL, like the LD Macintosh, is that they use the same skills as LD, which reduces the need for specific training in VL, while facilitating the training of residents in the management of the airway by LD. In addition, intubation can be recorded for post-event teaching.

The study by De Jong et al., from the Montpellier group, evaluated the McGrath MAC (Aircraft Medical, Edinburgh, Scotland), a VL with a Macintosh type spade that allows intubation using conventional or indirect direct laryngoscopy. The results reported by these authors are similar to other studies, noting that it is easier to visualize the glottis using VL and that fewer attempts are required to achieve intubation. However, although De Jong et al. showed a significant reduction in the incidence of difficult laryngoscopy and/or difficult intubation with VL McGrath MAC (4 vs. 16%) in ICU patients did not provide information on whether or not actual intubation time was shorter [51].

In ICU, where patients are often under a cardiorespiratory compromise, reducing the time the patient is without adequate ventilation/oxygenation is probably more important than the time it takes to visualize the glottis. In the study by Yeatts et al. was found that a shorter time was required to insert an ETT when a conventional direct laryngoscopy was performed [56]. In fact, in this study, an IL with Glidescope (Verathon Médico, Bothell, WA) was associated with prolonged intubation times in trauma patients, with a longer time of hypoxemia and a higher mortality in patients with traumatic brain injury [57]. These results coincide with those of the ICU study carried out by Griesdale et al., who found that intubation with Glidescope VL resulted in lower oxygen saturations [58].

In addition, the study by De Jong et al., from the Montpellier group, evaluated McGrath MAC, a *"mixed"* VL that can be used both to obtain direct and indirect laryngoscopy vision [51]. This prospective study showed that systematic use of a *"mixed"* VL, also termed *"combo VL"* or *"combined VL"*, for intubation within a process of quality improvement using an algorithm of airway management significantly reduced the incidence of difficult laryngoscopy and/or difficult intubation.

In the multivariate analysis, the use of a standard laryngoscope was an independent risk factor for difficult laryngoscopy and/or difficult intubation, as was the Mallampati III or IV score and the status of nonexpert operator. On the other hand, in the subgroup of patients with difficult intubation predicted by the MACOCHA score (**Figure 3**), the incidence of difficult

MACOCHA Score Calculation Worksheet	Points
- Factors related to patient	
Mallampati Score III or IV	5
Obstructive Sleep Apnoea Syndrome	2
Reduced Mobility of Cervical Spine	1
Limited Mouth Opening <3cm	1
- Factors related to pathology	
Coma	1
Severe Hypoxaemia (<80%)	1
- Factor related to operator	
Non Anaesthesiologist	1
Total	**12**

Sources: De Jong et al. 2014a; 2013b
M. Mallampati score III or IV
A. Apnoea Syndrome (obstructive)
C. Cervical spine limitation
O. Opening mouth <3cm
C. Coma
H. Hypoxia
A. Anaesthesiologist Non trained

Coded from 0 to 12
0 = easy
12 = very difficult

Figure 3. Macocha score.

intubation was much higher in the standard laryngoscope group (47%) than in the *"mixed"* VL group (0%). These results were in agreement with the previous studies [51].

Cameron et al. perform a study to evaluate the odds of first-attempt success with video laryngoscopy compared with direct laryngoscopy, using a propensity-matched analysis to reduce the risk of bias, for intubations performed in a medical ICU. They accomplish an analysis of prospectively collected data for 809 consecutive intubations performed between 2012 and 2014 in the ICU of an academic tertiary referral center that supports fellowship training programs in pulmonary and critical care medicine [59].

This study comparing video laryngoscopy with direct laryngoscopy as performed by nonanesthesiologist trainees in a medical ICU demonstrates improved first-attempt success associated with video laryngoscopy. Author's findings are clinically significant and consistent with other reports and meta-analyses. These results, in combination with the existing literature on the success of video laryngoscopy and the availability of video laryngoscopy in most academic medical ICUs, suggest that video laryngoscopy should be considered the primary method of laryngeal visualization for intubations performed in ICUs, where there is increased risk of intubation-related complications.

A 2014 meta-analysis found that, compared with direct laryngoscopy, videolaryngoscopy improved glottis view and first-attempt success for orotracheal intubation in ICU [10]. However, both randomized controlled trials (RCTs) and observational studies were included in that study, and evidence from RCTs was limited. In the past months, new RCTs have debated the application of videolaryngoscopy in airway management in ICU [60, 61]. Bing-Cheng Zhao et al. performs a meta-analysis of RCTs to evaluate the effects of video laryngoscopy on first-attempt success and complications related to intubation in ICU patients [50].

Four RCTs enrolling 678 patients were included [60–63], and compared with direct laryngoscopy, videolaryngoscopy did not significantly improve first-attempt success rate (RR 1.17, 95% CI 0.89–1.53). In videolaryngoscopy groups, poor glottis visualization was less common (RR 0.30, 95% CI 0.14–0.64), and incidence of esophageal intubation was lower (RR 0.31, 95% CI 0.11–0.90). However, videolaryngoscopy did not reduce the time for successful intubation and other outcomes, including severe hypoxemia, hypotension, mechanical ventilation duration, and ICU mortality.

Nonetheless, trial sequential analysis showed that the current evidence on the use of videolaryngoscopy is still inconclusive. The prima facie question is whether there may be a type H error due to an inadequate sample size, seeing that there already exists a trend favoring the use of videolaryngoscopy in relation to the primary outcome of successful first-attempt intubation. A previously published meta-analysis of nine studies by De Jong et al. demonstrated the superiority of videolaryngoscopy versus direct laryngoscopy with an odds ratio (OR) of 2.07 (95% CI 1.35–3.16) [10]. Significant heterogeneity exists in the forest plot (P test 73%) with appreciable differences between the operators from inexperienced medical students to critical care medicine experts [50]. Nonanaesthesiologist as operator has been validated to be a risk factor for difficulty in intubation in ICU [64]. The operator's training and experience in comparative studies is, in our opinion, a critical factor which influences reported differences among various intubation devices. Out of the four randomized trials included for the meta-analysis [50], data from Silverberg et al. [61] was excluded for the analysis of time for successful intubation on the grounds of high bias risk (due to suboptimal allocation concealment and randomization strategy). The study by Silverberg demonstrated statistically and clinically significant differences in the time for successful intubation favoring videolaryngoscopy. Non-inclusion may affect the pooled data analysis by Zhao et al. [50]. Curiously, data from the same study was included for pooled analysis of the primary outcome (rate of successful intubation on the first-attempt). Two of the included studies compared the performance of the Glidescope with direct laryngoscopy, and two pooled data sets were included from studies comparing the McGrath videolaryngoscope against direct laryngoscope. Not all videolaryngoscopes are the same and the airway literature distinguishes channeled videolaryngoscopes versus the anteriorly angulated variety versus the Macintosh-like videolaryngoscopes—appreciating peculiar advantages and disadvantages of each. Combining results from all videolaryngoscopes as an entity may have its limitations.

In this regard, Joshi et al. [65] have tried to identify characteristics associated with first-attempt failure at intubation when using videolaryngoscopy in the ICU. They perform an observational study of 906 consecutive patients intubated in the ICU with a video laryngoscope between January 2012 and January 2016 in a single-center academic medical ICU. After each intubation, the operator completed a data collection form, which included information on difficult airway characteristics, device used, and outcome of each attempt.

In this single-center study, there were no significant differences in sex, age, reason for intubation, or device used between first-attempt failures and first-attempt successes. First-attempt successes more commonly reported no difficult airway characteristics were present (23.9%; 95% confidence interval [CI], 20.7–27.0% vs. 13.3%, 95% CI, 8.0–18.8%).

Presence of blood in the airway (OR, 2.63, 95% CI, 1.64–4.20), airway edema (OR, 2.85; 95% CI, 1.48–5.45), and obesity (OR, 1.59, 95% CI, 1.08–2.32) were significantly associated with higher odds of first-attempt failure, when intubation was performed with videolaryngoscopy in an ICU.

In a second logistic model to examine cases in which these additional difficult airway characteristics were collected (n = 773), the presence of blood (OR, 2.73, 95% CI, 1.60–4.64), cervical immobility (OR, 3.34, 95% CI, 1.28–8.72), and airway edema (OR, 3.10; 95% CI, 1.42–6.70) were associated with first-attempt failure [65].

There are important limitations in this study, such that when certain difficult airway characteristics such as blood, vomit, or airway edema could have been known before the intubation attempt or encountered during the attempt, it is possible that operator reporting of these difficult airway characteristics was more common when they were unexpectedly encountered. Moreover, multivariable analyses account for experience of the operator. The generalization of these study results may be limited given the exposure, airway curriculum, and experience of trainees at this institution compared to others.

Nevertheless, the intensive care professional should account for these difficult airway characteristics, blood, cervical immobility, and airway edema, when preparing for endotracheal intubation with video laryngoscopy in addition to standard practices employed to optimize first-attempt success.

Janz et al. [62] evaluates the effect of video laryngoscopy on the rate of endotracheal intubation on first laryngoscopy attempt in a randomized, parallel-group, pragmatic trial of video compared with direct laryngoscopy among 150 critically ill adults undergoing endotracheal intubation by Pulmonary and Critical Care Medicine fellows in a Medical ICU in a tertiary, academic medical center.

The primary outcome was the rate of intubation on first-attempt, adjusted for the operator's previous experience with the intubating device at the time of the procedure. Adjustment for the operator's previous device experience was performed by collecting the number of times the operator had previously used a VL or DL at the time of each intubation event during the trial, such that the adjustment for prior experience with a specific device was updated constantly as the trial progressed.

Videolaryngoscopy improves glottic visualization but does not appear to increase procedural success in unadjusted analyses or after adjustment for the operator's previous experience with the assigned device (OR for video laryngoscopy on intubation on first-attempt 2.02, 95% CI, 0.82–5.02, p = 0.12). Secondary outcomes of time to intubation, lowest arterial oxygen saturation, complications, and in-hospital mortality were not different between video and direct laryngoscopy [62].

The results of all of these studies are in contrast with results of prior studies demonstrating improved procedural success with VL [30, 36, 61]. There are several potential explanations for this difference, as that prior study limited to noncritically ill populations [66] may not apply to the patient, operator, and procedural conditions surrounding intubation in the ICU.

A lack of accounting of the experience of the operator at the time of the procedure [30, 36, 49, 61, 67] may also confound the results all of these works.

Several studies have shown that videolaryngoscopy enhances the laryngeal view in patients with apparently normal and anticipated difficult airways [32, 33, 39, 53, 68–70]. And there are a number of possible reasons why improving glottis view with VL does not translate into procedural success. Therefore, these data may not be generalizable to operators using videolaryngoscopes other than the McGrath MAC and direct laryngoscopes with straight blades. And some authors theorize that improving glottic view with VL may only matter to less-experienced operators [62].

The MACMAN trial (McGrath Mac Videolaryngoscope Versus Macintosh Laryngoscope for Orotracheal Intubation in the Critical Care Unit) is a multicentre, open-label, randomized controlled superiority trial published in JAMA [63]. It was a multicenter, randomized, open-label trial, which included all ICU patients that needed orotracheal intubation.

Lascarrou et al. try to determine whether video laryngoscopy increases the frequency of successful first-pass orotracheal intubation compared with direct laryngoscopy in ICU patients. They perform a randomized clinical trial of 371 adults requiring intubation while being treated at 7 ICUs in France between 2015 and 2016, and there was 28 days of follow-up.

The primary outcome was the proportion of patients with successful first-pass intubation. The secondary outcomes included time to successful intubation and mild to moderate and severe life-threatening complications.

The first intubation attempts were made by a nonexpert in 83.8% of patients. There were no difference in first-pass success between the VL (67.7%) and the ML (70.3%) groups (absolute difference, −2.5% [95% CI, −11.9% to 6.9%]; p = 0.60. These results were sustained even after adjusting for operator expertise and MACOCHA score.

The proportion of first-attempt intubations performed by nonexperts (primarily residents, n = 290) did not differ between the groups (84.4% with videolaryngoscopy vs. 83.2% with direct laryngoscopy; absolute difference 1.2% [95% CI, −6.3% to 8.6%]; p = 0.76). The median time to successful intubation was 3 min (range, 2–4 min) for both videolaryngoscopy and direct laryngoscopy (absolute difference, 0 [95% CI, 0 to 0]; p = 0.95). Videolaryngoscopy was not associated with life-threatening complications (24/180 [13.3%] vs. 17/179 [9.5%] for direct laryngoscopy; absolute difference, 3.8% [95% CI, −2.7% to 10.4%]; p = 0.25). In post hoc analysis, videolaryngoscopy was associated with severe life-threatening complications (17/179 [9.5%] vs. 5/179 [2.8%] for direct laryngoscopy; absolute difference, 6.7% [95% CI, 1.8% to 11.6%]; p = 0.01) but not with mild to moderate life-threatening complications (10/181 [5.4%] vs. 14/181 [7.7%]; absolute difference, −2.3% [95% CI, −7.4% to 2.8%]; p = 0.37).

The main reason for intubation failure in the ML group was inability to see the glottis, and in the VL group was failure of tracheal catheterization.

The ability to see the glottis is related to the expertise with the procedure and the equipment you are using, either way, since the groups were balanced regarding the physicians' expertise, the difference found between the two groups here might be because it is easier to visualize the glottis with the VL. The failure of tracheal catheterization, 70.7% (VL) vs. 23.5% (ML), can be explain with the learning curve or because they study a non-channeled VL. Eye-hand coordination, especially when looking through a monitor, is not learned with a few training sessions. Stratified by center and *"the status of expertise or nonexpertise of the individual performing intubation"*. Unfortunately, the expert defying criteria did not include any experience with VL, and a good explanation for this difference is the lack of experience with the VL device besides the absence of channel in the blade.

Several studies comparing videolaryngoscopy with direct laryngoscopy have demonstrated improved rates of first-attempt success in the operating room, emergency department, trauma unit, and simulation laboratory, as well as during active cardiopulmonary resuscitation [56–58, 71–80]. Data comparing videolaryngoscopy with direct laryngoscopy on first-attempt success in the ICU are limited to a small number of observational studies [30, 36, 81–83], a meta-analysis of those studies [10], and some randomized controlled trials [60, 61].

Randomized controlled trial data comparing video laryngoscopy with direct laryngoscopy in the medical ICU are limited in number and external validity, especially for intubations performed by nonanesthesiologists.

6.4. Limitations

Videolaryngoscopes have among their disadvantages the cost, which mainly restriction access in areas outside the operating room. Devices need to be connected to the mains or batteries, and those that have an external monitor connected by cable may be little *"portable"*.

Because they provide an indirect image, the blood, secretions, and fogging of the lens obscure the image.

The fogging can be prevented by pre-aspirating the pharynx, or by preheating or applying specific solutions to the distal lens if the device does not have a concrete anti-fogging system (such as GlideScope, Airtraq, King Vision, etc.).

Like any other device, VLs require a learning curve. Those who have a shovel similar to that of the Macintosh (without a canal) need a transglottic device (guarantor, Frova, Eschman, etc.), inserted through a technique that must be learned since they can generate traumatisms on the soft palate during its introduction. On the other hand, if the operator cannot properly position the device-channel blade, the tube can be guided into the esophagus. When this occurs, while maintaining a good vision of the glottis and the patient remains stable and well oxygenated, we can try to solve the problem by a light movement of the device (**Figure 4**) or the ETT (**Figure 5**), which will help guide the ETT and achieve successful intubation.

6.5. Complications

All of these devices allow an optimal visualization of the glottic anatomy, but sometimes the maneuvers required for intubation involve greater complexity because of the difficulty in orienting the ETT.

For this reason, specific guides and catheters have been designed for intubation.

Nevertheless, in parallel with the clinical use of these devices, complications have been described.

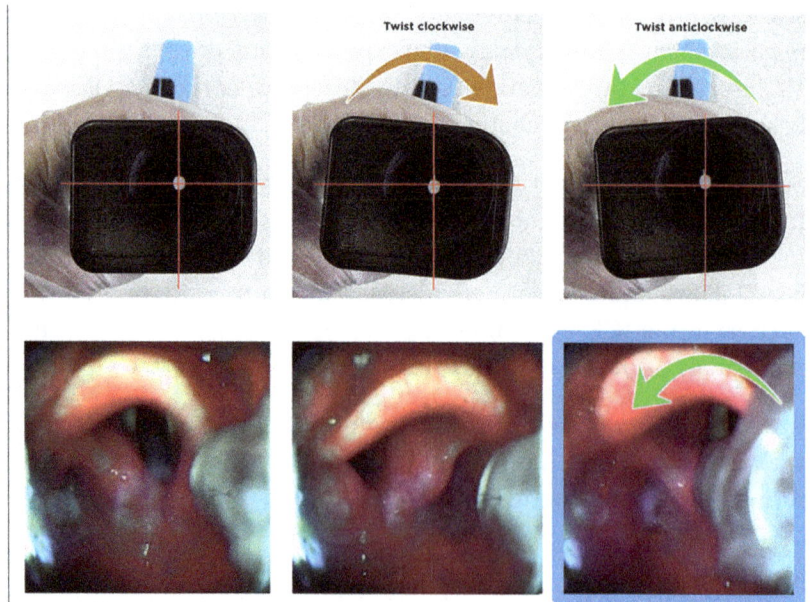

Figure 2. Technique to guide Endotracheal Tube (ETT)

Airtraq Turn

If the ETT initially touches the right side of the epiglottis or arytenoids, the Airtraq should be turned to orienting the vocal cords

In most cases, a small turn anticlockwise will assist in blowing the ETT

Twist clockwise

Twist anticlockwise

Figure 4. Technique to guide endotracheal tube (ETT).

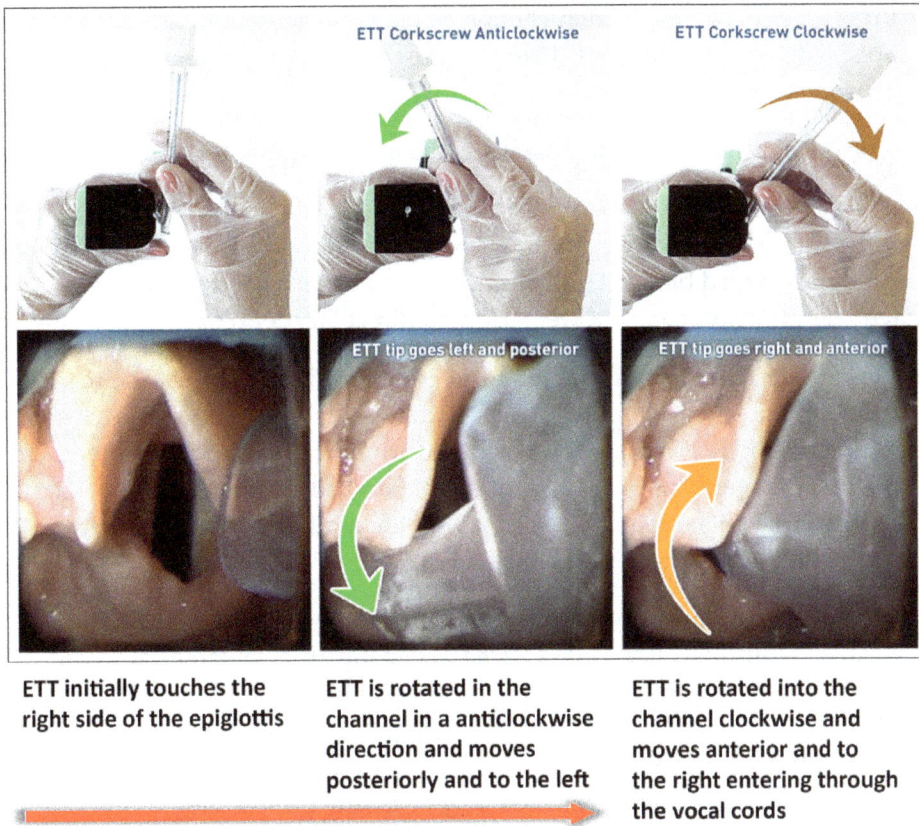

ETT initially touches the right side of the epiglottis

ETT is rotated in the channel in a anticlockwise direction and moves posteriorly and to the left

ETT is rotated into the channel clockwise and moves anterior and to the right entering through the vocal cords

Figure 5. Technique for orienting the endotracheal tube (ETT).

Thus, lacerations of the glottic mucosa, vocal cord lesions, subluxations of arytenoids, and supracarinal tears are some of the complications encountered with the use of these new devices.

6.6. Practical approach to videolaryngoscopy

If we decide to use any device in our patients we think about practical approach of this device and not only in theoretical applications. In the case of videolaryngoscopes, we can raise doubts about how is the procedure different of direct videolaryngoscopy?

When we will perform the intubation, we must take into account that videolaryngoscope intubation is quite different than traditional direct laryngoscopy. The videolaryngoscope blade must be inserted into the middle of the mouth and rotated around the tongue in order to line up the camera lens with the larynx.

Always insert the videolaryngoscope midline into the mouth looking at the patient until its tip has passed the palate.

Once the blade has turned the corner into the pharynx, look at the monitor while glancing at your patient to optimally position the blade.

There are three types of blade. The non-channeled blades can be equal to the traditional direct laryngoscope blade or can be angled. This angle used to be 60° or similar, and make impossible direct visualization of the glottis.

The third type is the channeled blades that have a channel to lead the ETT toward to the glottis.

We have to be very clear that videolaryngoscopes allow a view of the entrance of glottis independent of the line of sight, especially those that have angled blades, but if we use a non-channeled and non-angled blade, it will be equal to the traditional direct laryngoscope blade, and we have a similar glottic view if we perform a direct laryngoscopy.

Other important question is about patient head position regard. One of the most important features of these devices, particularly angled blades, is that the head and neck should be in extreme sniffing position or in a neutral position during all the intubation intent. We can see indirectly glottis, independent of the line of sight, because the image sensor is in the distal part of the blade. This give us a panoramic view of the glottis, without the need to "align the axes", thus avoiding hyperextension of the head.

But, if we do not need to move head's patient, do we still lift the jaw upward like in direct videolaryngoscopy? In clinical practice, Cormack-Lehane grade obtained with videolaryngoscopes use to be one or two at last in 99% of the cases. But, this view not guarantees the success of intubation, which is relatively frequent in videolaryngoscopes that have a curved leaf, especially during the learning stage. This difficulty in achieving intubation despite the correct exposure of the larynx even in expert hands may be finally impossible.

So, in practice, sometimes perform the traditional maneuvers as lift the jaw upward, BURP maneuver, wear the epiglottis or move carefully the videolaryngoscope can facilitate the intubation.

As stated above, usually all patients had grade 1 or 2 Cormack-Lehane views (grade 1: full glottic view; grade 2: partial glottic view; grade 3: epiglottis visible but no glottic view; and grade 4: epiglottis not visible) with videolaryngopscopes. However, achieving CL grade 1 laryngoscopy in videolaryngoscopy does not guarantee the success of OTI, which is relatively frequent in VLs that have a curved leaf.

There have been a number of maneuvers suggested to increase the success of passing the endotracheal tube when glottic visualization is excellent and the tube is not easily passed using usual methods.

With non-channeled blades, once the blade is positioned with the larynx in view (as we explain in the previous point), we insert the ETT along the right side of the blade. Even though the magnificent view of the larynx on the monitor at this point, we must remember that the larynx is not in the direct line of sight.

Therefore, a properly curved stylet must be used to guide the endotracheal tube into the larynx. Unlike the typical "hockey-stick" shape used during direct laryngscopy and in the standard videolaryngoscope blades, the stylet should match the curve on the angled blades.

If it is being used a standard stylet, it must be placed into the ETT and then mold it against the blade so that the curves match. The ETT can leave into the sleeve to keep it clean.

Because a standard disposable stylet is so malleable, occasionally it will straighten during insertion, especially if the oral space is tight. This leads to the scenario of being able to see the larynx and not being able to "get there". There are specific stylets, some of them nondisposable, which are preconfigured to the correct curve of their videolaryngoscope. Some of them are very stiff and can potentially damage pharyngeal structures, so that they must pull back slightly before fully inserting the ETT into the trachea.

Regardless of which stylet you are using, insert the endotracheal tube with the curve aimed toward the right side of the mouth, under direct vision until to see it on the monitor.

At this point rotate the tube back toward the midline, and aim it at the glottic opening.

If the mouth is small, it can be helpful to insert the ETT into the mouth first, slide it far to the right side of the mouth, and then insert the videolaryngoscope non-channeled blade midline.

To avoid lesions, it is mandatory to look at the patient during insertion of the ETT as described above until its tip has passed out of view beyond the tonsillar pillars. Only after the tip of the ETT has turned the corner into the pharynx should you look at the monitor, otherwise you can injure teeth, lips, tongue, and pharyngeal structures. Manipulate the tip of the tube through the glottis, and then pause to withdraw the stylet 2–3 cm. to effectively soften the tip of the ETT. Advance the ETT into the trachea looking at the monitor.

Channeled videolaryngoscopes have the advantage of orienting the ETT toward the trachea, allowing directed intubation with a little manipulation of the airway.

After successful intubation, remove the videolaryngoscope looking at the patient, not the monitor.

And, finally, we must think about regurgitation. Cricoid pressure, also named Sellick maneuver, is a standard anesthetic maneuver used to reduce the risk of aspiration of gastric contents during the induction of general anesthesia, applied after induction, in the period between loss of consciousness and placement of a cuffed tracheal tube. This is also a standard component of a rapid sequence induction technique. Cricoid pressure has been shown to prevent gastric distension during mask ventilation too.

A correct Sellick maneuver should be applied with a force of 10 N when the patient is awake, increasing to 30 N as consciousness is lost. These pressures occlude the esophagus and prevent aspiration during intubation, but often resulting in worsened glottis view and complicate intubation.

If initial attempts at videolaryngoscopy are difficult during rapid sequence induction, cricoid pressure should be released. This should be done under vision and suction available and, if we see regurgitation, cricoid pressure should be immediately reapplied.

7. Optimization of processes

In most cases, there is sufficient time to improve the intubation conditions, to perform an initial assessment and to evaluate the risk of intubation, to verify the availability of material, inductive agents and to plan alternatives.

Even so, on other occasions, the urgency of intubation in ICU is extreme (cardiorespiratory arrest, polytrauma, coma, etc.), and OTI should be performed in an optimal attempt of intubation with little time to optimize the patient.

Critical patient may present, mainly, hypoxemia, severe metabolic acidosis, hypotension, and right ventricular insufficiency [9, 16, 19, 20], with a degree of hemodynamic instability resulting in a low cardiopulmonary reserve, in addition to a full stomach, etc., and the implementation of a package of measures for intubation can reduce the incidence of life-threatening complications from 32 to 17% (p = 0.01) during intubation (biblioUCI46). This package of measures should consist of 10 key points (**Table 2**).

Of these recommendations, six have individually demonstrated their benefit, both in anesthetic practice and in critical care (noninvasive mechanical ventilation [NIM], the presence of two operators, rapid sequence intubation [drugs and Sellick maneuver], capnography, and protection ventilation pulmonary).

The presence of a second operator in crisis situations has been shown to reduce the complications associated with the OTI procedure such as esophageal intubation (0.9% vs. 3.4%), traumatic intubation (1.7% vs. 6.8%), bronchoaspiration (0.9% vs. 5.8%), tooth damage (0% vs. 1.0%), and selective intubation (2.6% vs. 7.2%). The overall rate of complications also decreased significantly (6.1% vs. 21.7%, p < 0.0001) [89].

Prior to intubation

1. Presence of two operators.

2. Perform a loading of fluids (500 ml of isotonic saline or 250 ml of colloid) in the absence of cardiopulmonary edema.

3. Preparation of maintenance sedation.

4. Preoxygenation for 3 min with noninvasive mechanical ventilation (NIMV) in case of acute respiratory failure (100% FiO_2, ventilatory support pressure between 5 and 15 cm H_2O, to obtain an expiratory volume between 6 and 8 ml kg^{-1} and a PEEP of 5 cm H_2O).

During intubation

Rapid sequence intubation (RSI): etomidate 0.2–0.3 mg kg^{-1} or ketamine 1.5–3 mg kg^{-1}, combined with succinylcholine 1–1.5 mg kg^{-1} in the absence of allergy, hyperkalemia, severe acidosis, acute or chronic neuromuscular disease, burn patient of more than 48 h evolution and spinal cord trauma. Rocuronium bromide (rocuronium) 0.9–1.2 mg kg^{-1} may be used when succinylcholine is not indicated [84–87].

5. *Sellick maneuver* [88].

Post-intubation

6. Immediate confirmation of the position of the ETT by *capnography*.

7. Noradrenaline if diastolic BP remains <35 mmHg.

8. Initiate long-term sedation.

9. Initiate *lung protection mechanical ventilation*: tidal volume 6–8 ml kg^{-1}. According to ideal weight, PEEP <5 cm H_2O, and respiratory frequency between 10 and 20 resp./min, FiO_2 100% for a plateau pressure <30 cm H_2O.

Table 2. Package of measures for intubation in ICU.

Therefore, prior to anesthetic induction, at least the presence of two operators, water overload and preoxygenation with NIMV is recommended for 3 min in case of acute respiratory failure.

7.1. Patient's preparation

Before the AM should be prepared the basic material:

- Ventilation: facial mask of adequate size, manual resuscitator, oropharyngeal cannula.

- Intubation: laryngoscopes, videolaryngoscopes, endotracheal tubes, extraglottic devices (such as FROVA or an introducer of Eschmann).

- Position: the position of the patient is an important factor and limits the reduction of functional residual capacity. Several studies have shown that prior oxygenation in the semi-seated position or with the head at 25° can achieve greater PaO_2 [90, 91].

- Vacuum cleaner.

- Medication.

In the case of expected intubation difficulty, there should be a practically immediate availability of advanced AM material with different rescue devices of ventilation and intubation difficulty, as well as a Coniotomy cannula in the event of an eventual CICO situation.

The ICU should have prepared a difficult airway trolley, similar to those that can be found in the surgical blocks [1] (**Figure 6**).

7.2. Preoxygenation

Acute hypoxemic insufficiency is the main cause of intubation in the ICU.

One-third of patients had severe arterial desaturation ($SatO_2 < 80\%$) during intuation manevers.

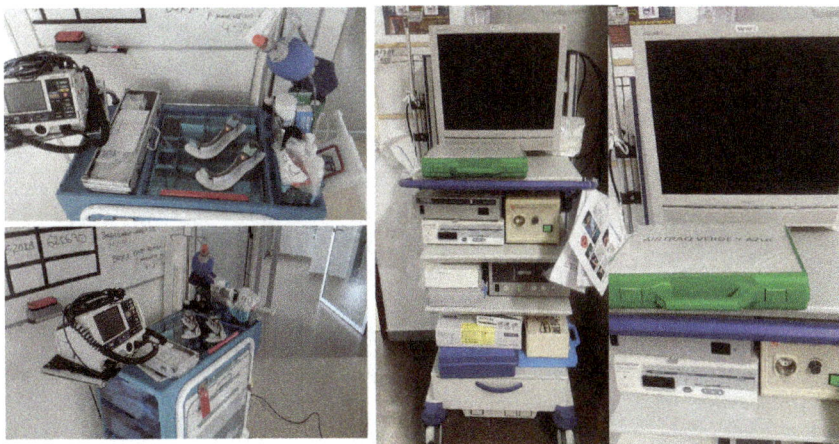

Figure 6. Reanimation difficult airway trolley examples. Left, Infanta Leonor University Hospital. Right, Getafe University Hospital, Madrid, Spain.

Hypoxemia may favor the complications observed during intubation such as arrhythmias, myocardial ischemia, cardiac arrest, and hypoxia in the brain.

Preoxygenation is the administration of 100% FiO_2 before induction. This maneuver aims to displace the alveolar nitrogen (N_2) by replacing it with oxygen (denitrogenation), in order to obtain an intrapulmonary O_2 reserve that allows the maximum apnea time with the lowest desaturation [92–96].

Traditional preoxygenation, performed with ventilation at current volume with Mapleson circuit and well-sealed facial mask, using a fresh gas flow of 5 L/min. of 100% oxygen for 3–5 min [94], is insufficient in the critical patient [97]. And only 50% of these patients will experience an increase of their PaO_2 higher than 5% compared to their baseline values after conventional preoxygenation for 4 min [98].

In all ICU patients, preoxygenation should be performed using a NIMV with PEEP 5–10 cm H_2O + PS 5–15 with FiO_2 100%, a management that has been shown to prevent patient desaturation during the procedure [98].

The mean pressure on AM will lead to alveolar recruitment, with the temporary reduction of intrapulmonary shunt [99] and an improvement in oxygenation. However, when this positive pressure is removed for OTI there is a risk of alveolar dis-reclusion, which will cause rapid desaturation.

Maintenance of continuous positive pressure during intubation with the use of a nasal mask has been shown to be beneficial in the operating room to patients with hypoxemic respiratory insufficiency and may be useful in ICU [100]. This apnea (or apneic) oxygenation is based on the alveolar pressure exerted by the blood circulation in the alveoli at slightly sub-atmospheric levels, generating a negative pressure gradient.

Another option is the high-flow nasal cannula (CNAF), a system that can provide up to 100% warm and humidified FiO_2 at a maximum flow of 60 L/min. [101].

This system allows an increase in CO_2 clearance due to better pharyngeal space clearance [102], in addition to the generation of a continuous positive pressure in flow-dependent AM (CPAP) (up to 7.4 cm H_2O to 60 L/min), with the reduction of respiratory resistance and maintenance of alveolar opening.

7.3. Recruitment maneuver

Idea of NIMV use during preoxygenation is to recruit lung tissue available for gas exchange: *"open the lung"* with PS, and *"keep the lung open"* with PEEP.

The combination of preoxygenation/denitrogenation (with FiO_2 100%) and the apneic period associated with the OTI procedure can dramatically decrease the pulmonary ventilation volume ratio, causing atelectasis.

Recruitment maneuver (RM) consists of a transient increase in inspiratory pressure, and there are several possible maneuvers such as applying a CPAP of 40 cm H_2O during 30–40 s immediately after the OTI. When compared with not do, RM is associated with a higher PaO_2 (with FiO_2 100%) 5 min (93 ± 36 vs. 236 ± 117 mmHg) and 30 min (39 ± 180 vs. 110 ± 79 mmHg) after intubation [103, 104].

7.4. Hypotension

Peri-OTI hypotension is a risk factor for adverse events, including cardiorespiratory arrest related to the management of AM, and up to 30% of critically ill patients may present post-OTI cardiovascular collapse [21, 54, 105–107].

Systolic blood pressure (SBP) <70 mmHg complicates 10% of intubations in ICU patients [9, 54, 106, 107], and when the patient has a preinduction gravity HR/SBP > 0.8, hemodynamic optimization should be performed pre-OTI and use inducing drugs with little response.

In responder patients, resuscitation with volume [108–110] can be made, while in the nonresponders, a perfusion of noradrenaline will be initiated [111, 112].

If pre-OTI resuscitation is not feasible due to the critical situation of the patient, vasoactive drugs will be prepared for bolus administration in order to maintain blood pressure during OTI and subsequent resuscitation. Although there is insufficient evidence, adrenaline diluted at a concentration of 1–10 mcg mL^{-1}, to be administered in boluses of 10–50 mcg, may be most indicated because of its inotropic effect [16, 109, 110, 113, 114].

In patients who are not in shock but exhibit a transient drop in post-OTI blood pressure due to the vasodilatory effects of induction agents or the onset of positive pressure ventilation, diluted phenylephrine at a concentration of 100 mcg mL^{-1} will be administered in boluses at 50–200 mcg [16, 109, 110].

7.5. Severe metabolic acidosis

When acidemia develops from respiratory acidosis, it can be corrected rapidly by increasing alveolar ventilation. However, when acidemia depends on metabolic acidosis, maintenance of acid-base homeostasis depends on compensatory respiratory alkalosis based on alveolar hyperventilation.

In situations of severe metabolic acidosis such as diabetic ketoacidosis, poisoning salicylate, or severe lactic acidosis, the patient may not be able to make an alveolar hyperventilation that achieves buffering generated organic acids with a worsening acidosis [9, 16, 19, 20, 105, 115].

When OTI is required in these patients, even a brief apnea time can lead to a significant drop in pH given the loss of respiratory compensation that was already insufficient.

Therefore, OTI should be avoided in patients with severe metabolic acidosis in whom adequate ventilation with the ventilator cannot be ensured, and NIV can be used to adequately support respiratory work until correction of underlying metabolic acidosis.

If the OTI cannot be delayed, getting the patient to maintain spontaneous ventilation becomes a critical action during intubation and mechanical ventilation, as this will allow the patient to maintain their own minute ventilation. For this, agents with a low probability of generating apnea should be used. In addition, rapid sequence intubation should be avoided if possible, and if deemed necessary, a short-acting neuromuscular blocker such as succinylcholine should be used.

Once OTI is achieved, a ventilator mode should be chosen that allows the patient to establish and maintain their own minute ventilation to maintain respiratory compensation better.

7.6. Right ventricular failure

The main function of the right ventricle and pulmonary circulation is gas exchange. Under normal conditions, these are a low pressure and high-volume system which, in addition, must dampen the dynamic changes in volume and blood flow resulting from breathing, positional changes, and changes in left ventricular cardiac output. The adaptations needed to meet these conflicting requirements result in reduced compensation capacity in the event of a rise in afterload or pressure [105, 113, 116].

The failure of the system generates right heart failure, so that the right ventricle becomes unable to meet the demands, dilating, retrograde flow, decreased coronary perfusion and, ultimately, systemic hypotension and cardiovascular collapse [107, 110, 117].

When a patient with right heart failure requires OTI, increased afterload and decreased preload associated with invasive mechanical ventilation often leads to this cardiovascular collapse [21, 54, 105, 107, 113, 118].

In these patients, we should try to achieve pre-OTI hemodynamic optimization, including reduction of afterload with inhaled pulmonary artery vasodilators such as inhaled nitric oxide (INO) [119] or inhaled epoprostenol (Flolan) [113, 120].

In addition, good preoxygenation due to the reduction of intrapulmonary shunt [99], as well as apneic oxygenation [98, 106] will be essential, as well as avoid hypercapnia and high alveolar pressures, because they lead to vasoconstriction.

8. Critical airway management algorithm

As in the surgical setting, in order to limit the incidence of serious complications during OTI in the ICU, the entire process (pre-, peri-, and post-intubation) should be guided by protocols oriented to patient safety [2, 46, 121–124].

This critical AM algorithm will be based, firstly, on the outcome of the assessment of the difficulty of intubation according to the MACOCHA score [51] (**Figure 7**).

Always check the availability of the equipment for the AM and an eventual DA before the OTI. And, in the case of desaturation <80% during the procedure, the patient will be ventilated.

In the case of failure of intubation and ventilation, emergency ventilation through NIMV through a SAD allowing intubation [125] will be performed.

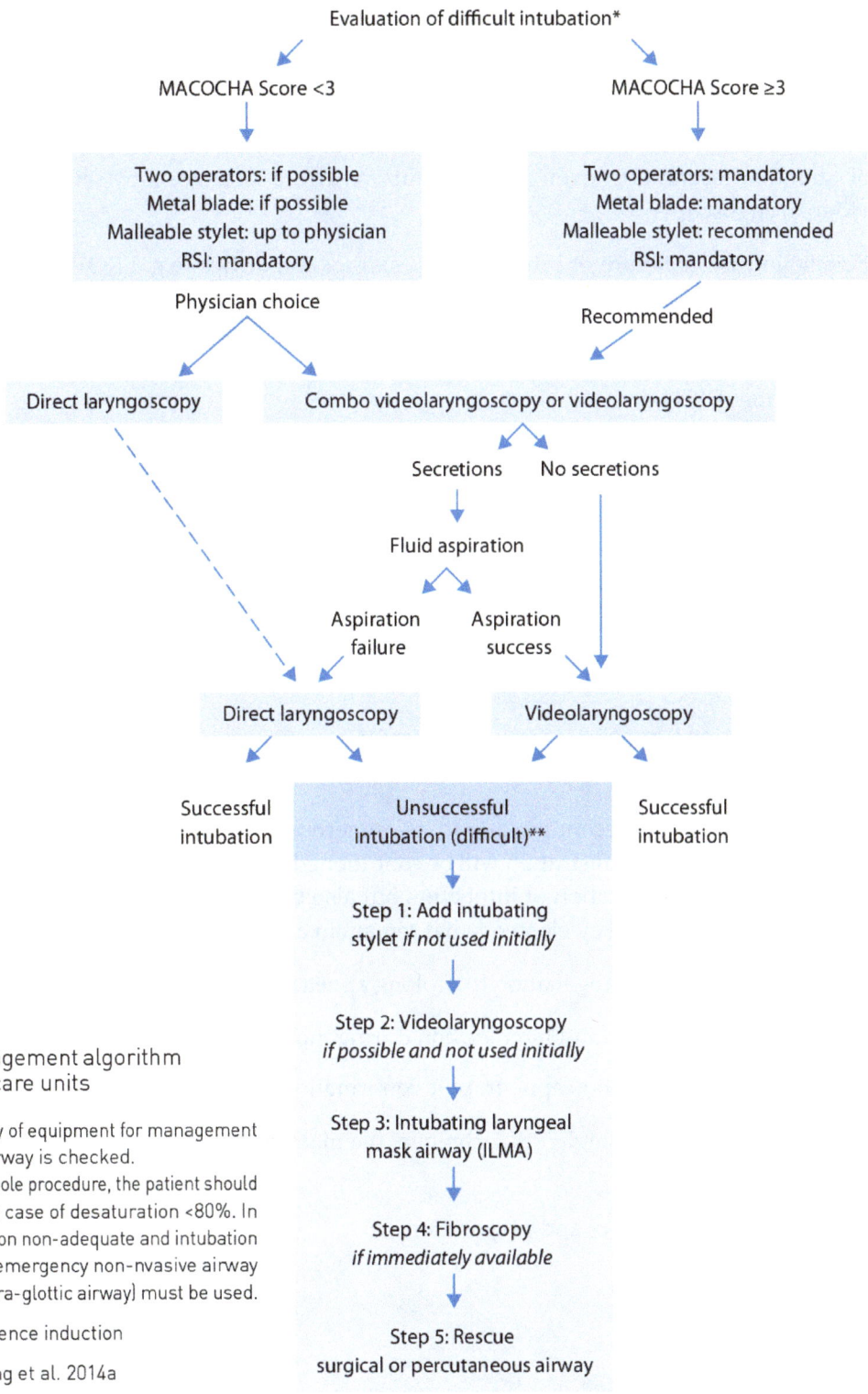

Evaluation of difficult intubation*

MACOCHA Score <3

MACOCHA Score ≥3

Two operators: if possible
Metal blade: if possible
Malleable stylet: up to physician
RSI: mandatory

Two operators: mandatory
Metal blade: mandatory
Malleable stylet: recommended
RSI: mandatory

Physician choice

Recommended

Direct laryngoscopy

Combo videolaryngoscopy or videolaryngoscopy

Secretions   No secretions

Fluid aspiration

Aspiration
failure

Aspiration
success

Direct laryngoscopy

Videolaryngoscopy

Successful
intubation

Unsuccessful
intubation (difficult)**

Successful
intubation

Step 1: Add intubating
stylet *if not used initially*

Step 2: Videolaryngoscopy
if possible and not used initially

Step 3: Intubating laryngeal
mask airway (ILMA)

Step 4: Fibroscopy
if immediately available

Step 5: Rescue
surgical or percutaneous airway

Airway management algorithm
in intensive care units

* The availability of equipment for management
of a difficult airway is checked.
** During the whole procedure, the patient should
be ventilated in case of desaturation <80%. In
case of ventilation non-adequate and intubation
unsuccessful, emergency non-nvasive airway
ventilation (supra-glottic airway) must be used.

RSI rapid sequence induction

Source: De Jong et al. 2014a

Figure 7. Macocha score protocol.

Two operators should always be present, especially if an AD with a MACOCHA score ≥3 is predicted, an extraglottic device (e.g. FROVA or an Eschmann introducer) should be used, and a rapid sequence induction be performed.

The use of a VL is also recommended in cases of difficult intubation. Nonetheless, in cases of abundant secretions, even after aspiration, direct laryngoscopy will be preferable to videolaryngoscopy.

Finally, in case of failure of intubation, an extraglottic device (e.g. FROVA or an Eschmann introducer) will be used first, followed by a VL if it was not initially used, rescue with a supraglottic airway device (SAD) that allows intubation, fiber optic bronchoscopy (FOB) and, at last, percutaneous or surgical rescue in situations of failure of intubation, ventilation, and oxygenation (CICO).

8.1. *"Not seemingly difficult"* airway management

It will be those patients who present a MACOCHA score <3.

The R rapid sequence induction (RSI) SI techniques are indicated in these cases, among others, in the ICU, hospital emergency services and out-of-hospital emergencies.

8.1.1. Rapid sequence intubation

The purpose of the RSI is to make emergency intubation easier and safer, and thus increase the success rate and reduce potential complications.

There is no single RSI technique due to its numerous indications, so the choice of the drug and the regimen of administration will be conditioned, not only by the reduction of the risk of aspiration and the facilitation of intubation but also by the characteristics of patient [88, 115, 126, 127]. However, the key elements that remain in all RSI protocol are:

• Preoxygenation/denitrogenation to prolong apnea time.

• Prevention of hypoxia and hypotension during induction and intubation.

• Use of a cuffed ETT, and capnographic confirmation of the placement of the tube.

In spite of the lack of a single RSI technique, the main steps could be summarized in [85, 88, 126, 127]:

• Valuation, planification, and preparation.

• Preoxygenation.

• Premedication.

• Induction and relaxation.

• Application of the Sellick maneuver.

• Laryngoscopy.

- Intubation. The RSI should allow us to intubate in a time no longer than 60 s from the administration of inducing drugs.

- Checking the placement of the ETT.

8.2. The anticipated difficult airway

Apnea following induction and neuromuscular relaxation may lead to rapid desaturation in the critical patient, if not in severe complications. In patients with previously DA [6, 40, 128, 129] or in those who were suspected according to a MACOCHA score ≥ 3, awake intubation would represent a valid option from the point of view of safety of the procedure [23, 29, 123, 130–133].

This intubation with the awake patient can be performed with a noninvasive technique or with an invasive technique (surgical or percutaneous), and among its advantages is that, by maintaining muscle tone, permeability of the airway and spontaneous ventilation, awake patients are easier to intubate because inducing general anesthesia tends to shift the larynx anterior.

The prerequisites for awake intubation in the ICU are:

- Previously difficult airway scenario or positive predictive signs (MACOCHA score ≥ 3).

- Patient cooperation.

- Equipment familiar with awake intubation techniques.

- Adequate AM preparation.

Contraindications:

- Human team inexperience.

- Negative of the patient.

- Allergy to local anesthetics.

- Hemorrhage in oropharyngeal cavity.

8.3. Difficult airway rescue

Before an intubation failure, we can find two possible scenarios:

- *Oxygenation with adequate face mask*: insisting repeatedly on a technique that has not resolved the situation will increase the risk of complications. Therefore, change to an alternative device (e.g. MCcoy blade), use an extraglottic device, use a VL, or a SAD intubation device.

- *Unsuitable oxygenation with face mask*: given the limited period of safe apnea of the critically ill patient, oxygenation, and not intubation, is the absolute priority in this scenario.

  There are different SAD that have been used to rescue ventilation with a difficult facial mask. The usual in ICU after ensuring oxygenation is that endotracheal intubation is necessary, so it is recommended to have some of the SAD that allow intubation through it [3].

  In the case of failure, a CICO scenario will be declared, the worst of the possible scenarios.

8.4. Can't-intubate-Can't-oxygenate scenario

CICO scenario is the end of the algorithms, and always constitutes a medical emergency that forces to explore an alternative plan based on transtracheal access, either through a percutaneous cricothyrotomy (choice for its speed), a surgical tracheotomy or through retrograde intubation.

This situation is reached when the attempt to AM had failed through tracheal intubation, facial mask ventilation, and a SAD. At this point, if the situation is not resolved quickly, hypoxic brain damage and death will occur.

The key points of the non-intubatable/non-oxygenable AM plan are:

• The CICO scenario must be declared and proceed to anterior neck access.

• A didactic technique has been described using a scalpel to promote standardized training.

• Placing an endotracheal balloon tube through the cricothyroid membrane facilitates normal minute ventilation with a standard ventilation system.

• High-pressure oxygenation through a fine cannula is associated with increased morbidity.

• All operators must be trained in performing a surgical approach.

• Training should be repeated at regular intervals to ensure that skills are not lost.

8.5. Adequate staff—adequate material—adequate procedure

Through the training program of those specialists who develop their professional activity in ICU must be guaranteed the acquisition of skills in critical patient's advanced airway management (**Figure 8**).

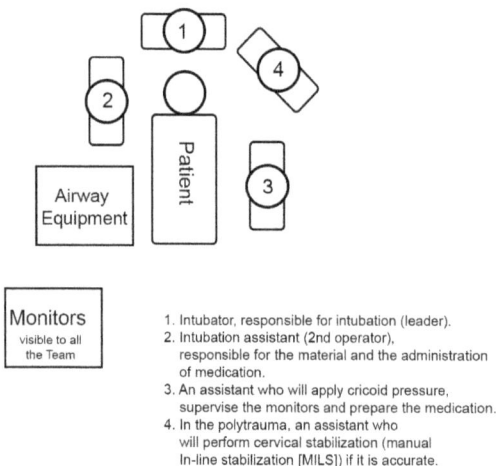
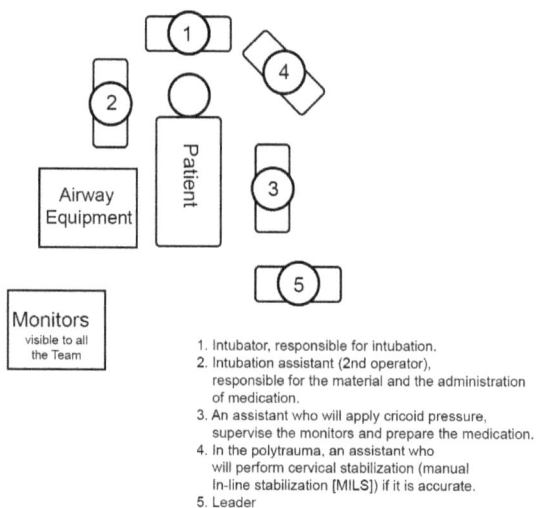

Figure 8. Teamwork, roles, goals and communication.

Those responsible for the training of each service should develop training programs based on simulation to maintain competencies with different devices: direct laryngoscopy, extraglottic devices, supraglottic devices, videolaryngoscopes, fiber optic bronchoscopes and cricothyrotomy set.

Also, each ICU should have immediate access 24 h a day to a difficult airway trolley that must include the same devices that the one usually available in the operating room.

9. Conclusions

Tracheal intubation in the critical patient is always potentially dangerous. Critically ill patients with acute respiratory, neurological, or cardiovascular failure requiring invasive mechanical ventilation are at high risk of difficult intubation and have organ dysfunctions associated with complications of intubation and anesthesia such as hypotension and hypoxemia. The complication rate increases with the number of intubation attempts. Videolaryngoscopy improves elective endotracheal intubation.

Every professional in ICU should have a basic knowledge about airway management, be familiar with algorithms to handle possible complications, and know correct use and interpretation of capnography. The algorithms that are usually handled by anesthesiologists in our routine clinical practice are not always useful in ICU because they contemplate alternatives such as awakening the patient or postponing the procedure that cannot be applied in a critical/emergency situation. The implementation of an intubation protocol in the ICU can contribute to significantly reduce the immediate severe complications associated with this procedure.

Airway management of patients admitted to the ICU is a challenge. New videolaryngoscopes have been proposed to improve management, but most studies comparing videolaryngoscopes with a standard direct laryngoscope (DL) have been performed in operating rooms. Therefore, the role of videolaryngoscopy in the ICU is still discussed, where there is a lack of scientific evidence and intubation conditions are worse than in the operating room. The Montpellier group has proposed and implemented a package for intubation care in its ICU which includes, among others, the use of two operators, fluid overload, preoxygenation, and, above all, the rapid detection of the position of the ETT by capnography. Including the use of videolaryngoscopy in this package, as described by De Jong et al. [51], the safety of tracheal intubation could be further improved.

The overall impact of VL on the anesthetic literature is weighed due to marked heterogeneity in the patient population, devices studied, operator experience, and confusion including manikin studies. While VL improves the ease of obtaining a view of the larynx, insertion of the ETT may be more difficult. VL may reduce the number of failed intubations, particularly among patients presenting with a difficult airway. They improve the glottic view and may reduce laryngeal/airway trauma. Currently, no evidence indicates that use of a VL reduces the number of intubation attempts or the incidence of hypoxia or respiratory complications, and no evidence indicates that use of a VL affects the time required for intubation [134].

The study of VL in the ICU is difficult for similar reasons, although they are increasing in popularity [10, 36]. However, there is a need for randomized controlled trials (RCTs) of VL vs. DL in the ICU [31], the truth is that the use of VL in ICU is so widespread that such studies are impractical. A RCT could help determine which devices are most useful, and could study the impact of VL on both technical and human factors [135].

If randomized controlled trials demonstrating a benefit of videolaryngoscopy are designed in the future, it could become a new standard for tracheal intubation in the ICU, particularly in educational institutions, where tracheal intubations are often performed by residents in training.

Nevertheless, the introduction of videolaryngoscopy in the ICU should always be accompanied by formal training programs in the management of the DA and simulation using manikins with the specific device [47, 71, 121, 136, 137].

Best way to avoid the serious consequences associated with a DA is the constant preparation by all those who could be able to handle it, an adequate prior assessment of the patient and the capacity to face this situation with the different rescue alternatives, from the use of SAD, VL, and flexibility in the use of the FOB, to the management of cervical surgical neck access.

Finally, we must implement the capnography in the ICU, so that the capnograph will be used in every intubation maneuver in the critical patient. Capnography should be monitored continuously in all critical intubated patients requiring assisted ventilation, and all ICU staff should be trained in the interpretation and recognition of abnormal capnography tracings.

In summary, if we consider the latest data, exclusive use of VL in out-of-OR airway management, or disdain them, appears premature, and we agree with the authors that future research would be necessary to demonstrate the safe utility of videolaryngoscopy in the ICU context. Even though it is surely the future to follow.

Author details

Eugenio Martinez Hurtado[1]*, Miriam Sanchez Merchante[2], Sonia Martin Ventura[3], Maria Luisa Mariscal Flores[3] and Javier Ripolles Melchor[1]

*Address all correspondence to: eugeniodaniel.martinez@salud.madrid.org

1 Department of Anaesthesia, Intensive Care Medicine and Pain Medicine, Hospital Universitario Infanta Leonor, Madrid, España

2 Department of Anaesthesia, Intensive Care Medicine and Pain Medicine, Hospital Universitario Fundación Alcorcón, Madrid, España

3 Department of Anaesthesia, Intensive Care Medicine and Pain Medicine, Hospital Universitario de Getafe, Madrid, España

References

[1] Cook TM, Woodall N, Harper J, Benger J. Major complications of airway management in the UK: Results of the Fourth National Audit Project of the Royal College of Anaesthetists and the Difficult Airway Society. Part 2: Intensive care and emergency departments. British Journal of Anaesthesia. 2011 May;**106**(5):632-642

[2] Apfelbaum JL, Hagberg CA, Caplan RA, Blitt CD, Connis RT, Nickinovich DG, et al. Practice guidelines for management of the difficult airway. Anesthesiology [Internet]. 2003 [cited 2017 Aug 2];**98**(2):1269-1277. Available from: http://anesthesiology.pubs. asahq.org/Article.aspx?doi=10.1097/ALN.0b013e31827773b2

[3] Frerk C, Mitchell VS, McNarry AF, Mendonca C, Bhagrath R, Patel A, et al. Difficult Airway Society 2015 guidelines for management of unanticipated difficult intubation in adults. British Journal of Anaesthesia [Internet]. 2015 Dec 1 [cited 2017 Aug 7];**115**(6):827-848. Available from: https://academic.oup.com/bja/article-lookup/doi/10.1093/bja/aev371

[4] Rose DK, Cohen MM. The airway: Problems and predictions in 18,500 patients. Canadian Journal of Anesthesia [Internet]. 1994 May [cited 2017 Aug 7];**41**(5):372-383. Available from: http://link.springer.com/10.1007/BF03009858

[5] El-Ganzouri AR, McCarthy RJ, Tuman KJ, Tanck EN, Ivankovich AD. Preoperative airway assessment. Anesthesia & Analgesia [Internet]. 1996 Jun [cited 2017 Aug 7];**82**(6):1197-1204. Available from: http://www.ncbi.nlm.nih.gov/pubmed/8638791

[6] Krage R, Van Rijn C, Van Groeningen D, Loer SA, Schwarte LA, Schober P. Cormack-Lehane classification revisited. British Journal of Anaesthesia [Internet]. 2010 Dec 1 [cited 2017 Aug 2];**105**(2):220-227. Available from: http://www.ncbi.nlm.nih.gov/pubmed/21081683

[7] Frost PJ, Hingston CD, Wise MP. Reducing complications related to endotracheal intubation in critically ill patients. Intensive Care Medicine [Internet]. 2010 Feb [cited 2017 Aug 7];**36**(8):1438. Available from: http://www.ncbi.nlm.nih.gov/pubmed/7856895

[8] Le Tacon S, Wolter P, Rusterholtz T, Harlay M, Gayol S, Sauder P, et al. Complications des intubations trachéales difficiles dans un service de réanimation médicale. Annales Françaises d'Anesthésie et de Réanimation [Internet]. 2000 Dec [cited 2017 Aug 7];**19**(10):719-724. Available from: http://www.ncbi.nlm.nih.gov/pubmed/11200758

[9] Griesdale DEG, Bosma TL, Kurth T, Isac G, Chittock DR. Complications of endotracheal intubation in the critically ill. Intensive Care Medicine [Internet]. 2008 Oct 5 [cited 2017 Aug 2];**34**(10):1835-1842. Available from: http://www.ncbi.nlm.nih.gov/pubmed/18604519

[10] De Jong A, Molinari N, Conseil M, Coisel Y, Pouzeratte Y, Belafia F, et al. Video laryngoscopy versus direct laryngoscopy for orotracheal intubation in the intensive care unit: A systematic review and meta-analysis. Intensive Care Medicine [Internet]. 2014 [cited 2017 Aug 2];**40**(5):629-639. Available from: http://link.springer.com/10.1007/s00134-014-3236-5

[11] Law JA, Broemling N, Cooper RM, Drolet P, Duggan LV, Griesdale DE, et al. The difficult airway with recommendations for management—Part 1—Intubation encountered in an unconscious/induced patient. Canadian Journal of Anesthesia [Internet]. 2013 Nov 17 [cited 2017 Aug 7];60(11):1089-1118. Available from: http://www.ncbi.nlm.nih.gov/pubmed/24132407

[12] Law JA, Broemling N, Cooper RM, Drolet P, Duggan LV, Griesdale DE, et al. The difficult airway with recommendations for management—Part 2—The anticipated difficult airway Prise en charge des voies aériennes—2e partie—Recommandations lorsque des difficultés sont prévues. Canadian Journal of Anesthesia [Internet]. 2013 Nov 17 [cited 2017 Aug 7];60(11):1119-1138. Available from: http://link.springer.com/10.1007/s12630-013-0020-x

[13] Han R, Tremper KK, Kheterpal S, O'Reilly M. Grading scale for mask ventilation. Anesthesiology [Internet]. 2004 Jul [cited 2017 Aug 7];101(1):267. Available from: http://www.ncbi.nlm.nih.gov/pubmed/15220820

[14] Kheterpal S, Han R, Tremper KK, Shanks A, Tait AR, O'Reilly M, et al. Incidence and predictors of difficult and impossible mask ventilation. Anesthesiology [Internet]. 2006 Nov [cited 2017 Aug 7];105(5):885-891. Available from: http://www.ncbi.nlm.nih.gov/pubmed/17065880

[15] Kheterpal S, Martin L, Shanks AM, et al. Prediction and outcomes of impossible mask ventilation. Anesthesiology [Internet]. 2009 Apr [cited 2017 Aug 7];110(4):891-897. Available from: http://www.ncbi.nlm.nih.gov/pubmed/19293691

[16] Mosier JM, Joshi R, Hypes C, Pacheco G, Valenzuela T, Sakles JC. The physiologically difficult airway. Western Journal of Emergency Medicine [Internet]. 2015 Dec 17 [cited 2017 Aug 2];16(7):1109-1117. Available from: http://www.ncbi.nlm.nih.gov/pubmed/26759664%5Cnhttp://www.pubmedcentral.nih.gov/articlerender.fcgi?artid=PMC4703154

[17] Huitink JM, Bouwman RA. The myth of the difficult airway: Airway management revisited. Anaesthesia [Internet]. 2015 Mar [cited 2017 Aug 7];70(3):244-249. Available from: http://doi.wiley.com/10.1111/anae.12989

[18] Hung O, Murphy M. Context-sensitive airway management. Anesthesia & Analgesia [Internet]. 2010 Apr 1 [cited 2017 Aug 7];110(4):982-983. Available from: http://www.ncbi.nlm.nih.gov/pubmed/20357142

[19] Mosier JM, Law JA. Airway management in the critically ill. Intensive Care Medicine. 2014;40(5):727-729

[20] Griesdale DEG, Henderson WR, Green RS. Airway management in critically ill patients. Lung. 2011;189(3):181-192

[21] Mort TC. The incidence and risk factors for cardiac arrest during emergency tracheal intubation: A justification for incorporating the ASA Guidelines in the remote location. Journal of Clinical Anesthesia. 2004;16(7):508-516

[22] Sakles JC, Chiu S, Mosier J, Walker C, Stolz U. The importance of first pass success when performing orotracheal intubation in the emergency department. Academic Emergency Medicine. 2013;**20**(1):71-78

[23] Thomas AN, McGrath BA. Patient safety incidents associated with airway devices in critical care: A review of reports to the UK National Patient Safety Agency. Anaesthesia. 2009;**64**(4):358-365

[24] Miguel-Montanes R, Hajage D, Messika J, Bertrand F, Gaudry S, Rafat C, et al. Use of high-flow nasal cannula oxygen therapy to prevent desaturation during tracheal intubation of intensive care patients with mild-to-moderate hypoxemia. Critical Care Medicine [Internet]. 2014;**43**(c):1-10. Available from: http://www.ncbi.nlm.nih.gov/pubmed/25479117

[25] Kabrhel C, Thomsen TW, Setnik GS, Walls RM. Orotracheal intubation. Nejm [Internet]. 2007 [cited 2017 Aug 2];**356**(Anestesia, urgencias):1-3. Available from: http://www.nejm.org/doi/abs/10.1056/NEJMvcm063574

[26] Cooke H. Laryngoscopy: Time to change our view. Anaesthesia [Internet]. 2009 Apr [cited 2017 Aug 7];**64**(10):1143-1144. Available from: http://www.ncbi.nlm.nih.gov/pubmed/19317697

[27] Berthelsen PG, Cronqvist M. The first intensive care unit in the world: Copenhagen 1953. Acta Anaesthesiologica Scandinavica [Internet]. 2003 Nov [cited 2017 Aug 8];**47**(10):1190-1195. Available from: http://www.ncbi.nlm.nih.gov/pubmed/14616314

[28] Kelly FE, Fong K, Hirsch N, Nolan JP. Intensive care medicine is 60 years old: The history and future of the intensive care unit. Clinical Medicine (Northfield Il) [Internet]. 2014 Aug 1 [cited 2017 Aug 8];**14**(4):376-379. Available from: http://www.ncbi.nlm.nih.gov/pubmed/25099838

[29] Flavin K, Hornsby J, Fawcett J, Walker D. Structured airway intervention improves safety of endotracheal intubation in an intensive care unit. British Journal of Hospital Medicine (Lond) [Internet]. 2012 Jun [cited 2017 Aug 7];**73**(6):341-344. Available from: http://www.ncbi.nlm.nih.gov/pubmed/22875325

[30] Kory P, Guevarra K, Mathew JP, Hegde A, Mayo PH. The impact of video laryngoscopy use during urgent endotracheal intubation in the critically ill. Anesthesia & Analgesia [Internet]. 2013 Jul [cited 2017 Aug 7];**117**(1):144-149. Available from: http://www.ncbi.nlm.nih.gov/pubmed/23687228

[31] Larsson A, Dhonneur G. Videolaryngoscopy: Towards a new standard method for tracheal intubation in the ICU? Intensive Care Medicine [Internet]. 2013 Dec 12 [cited 2017 Aug 2];**39**(12):2220-2222. Available from: http://link.springer.com/10.1007/s00134-013-3118-2

[32] Bradbury CL, Hillermann C, Mendonca C, Danha R. Analysis of the learning curve with the C-MAC video laryngoscope: A manikin study. Journal of Anesthesia & Clinical Research [Internet]. 2011;**2**(10):167. Available from: https://www.omicsonline.org/peer-reviewed/analysis-of-the-learning-curve-with-the-cmac-video-laryngoscope-a-manikin-study-2124.html

[33] Falcetta S, Pecora L, Orsetti G, Gentili P, Rossi A, Gabbanelli V, et al. The bonfils fiber-scope: A clinical evaluation of its learning curve and efficacy in difficult airway management. Minerva Anestesiologica [Internet]. 2012 Feb [cited 2017 Aug 7];**78**(2):176-184. Available from: http://www.ncbi.nlm.nih.gov/pubmed/22095109

[34] Greaves JD. Training time and consultant practice. British Journal of Anaesthesia. 2005;**95**(5):581-583

[35] Nouruzi-Sedeh P, Schumann M, Groeben H. Laryngoscopy via Macintosh blade versus GlideScope: Success rate and time for endotracheal intubation in untrained medical personnel. Anesthesiology [Internet]. 2009 Jan [cited 2017 Aug 7];**110**(1):32-37. Available from: http://anesthesiology.pubs.asahq.org/Article.aspx?doi=10.1097/ALN.0b013e318190b6a7

[36] Mosier JM, Whitmore SP, Bloom JW, Snyder LS, Graham LA, Carr GE, et al. Video laryngoscopy improves intubation success and reduces esophageal intubations compared to direct laryngoscopy in the medical intensive care unit. Critical Care [Internet]. 2013 Dec 3 [cited 2017 Aug 7];**17**(5):R237. Available from: http://ccforum.com/content/17/5/R237

[37] Karalapillai D, Darvall J, Mandeville J, Ellard L, Graham J, Weinberg L. A review of video laryngoscopes relevant to the intensive care unit. Indian Journal of Critical Care Medicine [Internet]. 2014 Jul [cited 2017 Aug 7];**18**(1):442-452. Available from: http://www.ncbi.nlm.nih.gov/pubmed/25097357

[38] Healy DW, Maties O, Hovord D, Kheterpal S. A systematic review of the role of video-laryngoscopy in successful orotracheal intubation. BMC Anesthesiology [Internet]. 2012 Dec 14 [cited 2017 Aug 7];**12**(1):32. Available from: http://bmcanesthesiol.biomedcentral.com/articles/10.1186/1471-2253-12-32%5Cnhttp://www.pubmedcentral.nih.gov/articlerender.fcgi?artid=3562270&tool=pmcentrez&rendertype=abstract

[39] Kaplan MB, Ward DS, Berci G. A new video laryngoscope-an aid to intubation and teaching. Journal of Clinical Anesthesia. 2002;**14**(8):620-626

[40] Hurtado EM, Pablo EL, Merchante MS, Flores MLM, Melchor JR, Cabezon NDL. Video-laryngoscopy Data Record. A Reality That Is Possible. 2015. Unpublished

[41] Hurtado EM, Merchante MS. Commentary to "Hemodynamic response to endotracheal intubation using C-Trach assembly and direct laryngoscopy". Saudi Journal of Anaesthesia. 2016 Oct-Dec;**10**(4):485-486.

[42] Eugenio Martínez Hurtado. Videolaringoscopios: Manual de actualizacion en Dispositivos Opticos [Internet]. 1st ed. Createspace Independent Publishing Platform, editor. Createspace Independent Publishing Platform; Edición: 1. ES; 2015. Available from: https://www.amazon.es/Videolaringoscopios-Manual-actualizacion-Dispositivos-Opticos/dp/1508874344/ref=sr_1_7?ie=UTF8&qid=1492155738&sr=8-7&keywords=eugenio+martinez+hurtado

[43] Pott LM, Murray WB. Review of video laryngoscopy and rigid fiberoptic laryngoscopy. Current Opinion in Anaesthesiology [Internet]. 2008 Dec [cited 2017 Aug 7];**21**(6):750-758. Available from: http://www.ncbi.nlm.nih.gov/pubmed/18997526

[44] Niforopoulou P, Pantazopoulos I, Demestiha T, Koudouna E, Xanthos T. Video-laryngoscopes in the adult airway management: A topical review of the literature. Acta Anaesthesiologica Scandinavica [Internet]. 2010 Oct [cited 2017 Aug 7];**54**(9):1050-1061. Available from: http://doi.wiley.com/10.1111/j.1399-6576.2010.02285.x

[45] Asai T. Videolaryngoscopes. Anesthesiology [Internet]. 2012 Mar [cited 2017 Aug 7];**116**(3): 515-517. Available from: http://anesthesiology.pubs.asahq.org/Article.aspx?doi=10.1097/ALN.0b013e318246e866

[46] Hurtado EM, Merchante MS, Flóres MLM, Saldaña PM, Escoda NA, Vecino JMC. Implantación de la Videolaringoscopia en la Historia Clínica Digital. 2015. Unpublished

[47] Manejo de la Via Aerea Evidencia Actual [Internet]. CreateSpace Independent Publishing Platform; Edición: 1. ES; 2017. Available from: https://www.amazon.es/Manejo-Via-Aerea-Evidencia-Actual/dp/1519140010/ref=sr_1_1?ie=UTF8&qid=1492155738&sr=8-1&keywords=eugenio+martinez+hurtado

[48] Hurtado EM, Merchante S, Melchor JR, Escoda NA, Cabezon NL, Saldaña PM. How Do We Face The Difficult Airway In Our Daily Practice? An International Survey. 2015. Unpublished

[49] Van Zundert A, Pieters B, Doerges V, Gatt S. Videolaryngoscopy allows a better view of the pharynx and larynx than classic laryngoscopy. British Journal of Anaesthesia [Internet]. 2012 Dec 1 [cited 2017 Aug 8];**109**(6):1014-1015. Available from: http://www.ncbi.nlm.nih.gov/pubmed/23154957

[50] Zhao BC, Huang TY, Liu KX. Video laryngoscopy for ICU intubation: A meta-analysis of randomised trials. Intensive Care Medicine [Internet]. 2017 Jun 4 [cited 2017 Aug 7];**43**(6):947-948. Available from: http://www.ncbi.nlm.nih.gov/pubmed/28260161

[51] De Jong A, Clavieras N, Conseil M, Coisel Y, Moury PH, Pouzeratte Y, et al. Imple-mentation of a combo videolaryngoscope for intubation in critically ill patients: A before-after comparative study. Intensive Care Medicine [Internet]. 2013 [cited 2017 Aug 2];**39**(12):2144-2152. Available from: http://link.springer.com/10.1007/s00134-013-3099-1

[52] Cook T, Behringer EC, Benger J. Airway management outside the operating room: Hazardous and incompletely studied. Current Opinion in Anaesthesiology [Internet]. 2012 Aug [cited 2017 Aug 7];**25**(4):461-469. Available from: http://dx.doi.org/10.1097/ACO.0b013e32835528b1%5Cnhttp://search.ebscohost.com/login.aspx?direct=true&AuthType=ip,url,cookie,uid&db=mdc&AN=22673785&site=ehost-live

[53] Butchart AG, Young P. The learning curve for videolaryngoscopy. Anaesthesia [Internet]. 2010 Nov [cited 2017 Aug 7];**65**(11):1145-1146. Available from: http://www.ncbi.nlm.nih.gov/pubmed/20946399

[54] Perbet S, De Jong A, Delmas J, Futier E, Pereira B, Jaber S, et al. Incidence of and risk factors for severe cardiovascular collapse after endotracheal intubation in the ICU: A multicenter observational study. Critical Care [Internet]. 2015 Dec 18 [cited 2017 Aug 7];**19**(1):257. Available from: http://www.pubmedcentral.nih.gov/articlerender.fcgi?artid=4495680&tool=pmcentrez&rendertype=abstract

[55] De Jong A, Jung B, Jaber S. Intubation in the ICU: We could improve our practice. Critical Care [Internet]. 2014 Mar 18 [cited 2017 Aug 7];**18**(2):209. Available from: http://ccforum.com/content/18/2/209%5Cnpapers3://publication/doi/10.1186/cc13776

[56] Yeatts DJ, Dutton RP, Hu PF, Chang Y-WW, Brown CH, Chen H, et al. Effect of video laryngoscopy on trauma patient survival: A randomized controlled trial. Journal of Trauma and Acute Care Surgery [Internet]. 2013 Aug [cited 2017 Aug 7];**75**(2):212-219. Available from: http://www.ncbi.nlm.nih.gov/pubmed/23823612

[57] Taylor AM, Peck M, Launcelott S, Hung OR, Law JA, MacQuarrie K, et al. The McGrath® Series 5 videolaryngoscope vs the Macintosh laryngoscope: A randomised, controlled trial in patients with a simulated difficult airway. Anaesthesia [Internet]. 2013 Feb [cited 2017 Aug 8];**68**(2):142-147. Available from: http://www.ncbi.nlm.nih.gov/pubmed/23121470

[58] Malik MA, Subramaniam R, Maharaj CH, Harte BH, Laffey JG. Randomized controlled trial of the Pentax AWS®, Glidescope®, and Macintosh laryngoscopes in predicted difficult intubation. British Journal of Anaesthesia [Internet]. 2009 Nov 1 [cited 2017 Aug 8];**103**(5):761-768. Available from: http://www.ncbi.nlm.nih.gov/pubmed/19783539

[59] Hypes CD, Stolz U, Sakles JC, Joshi RR, Natt B, Malo J, et al. Video laryngoscopy improves odds of first-attempt success at intubation in the intensive care unit a propensity-matched analysis. Annals of the American Thoracic Society [Internet]. 2016 Mar [cited 2017 Aug 8];**13**(3):382-389. Available from: http://www.ncbi.nlm.nih.gov/pubmed/26653096

[60] Griesdale DEG, Chau A, Isac G, Ayas N, Foster D, Irwin C, et al. Video-laryngoscopy versus direct laryngoscopy in critically ill patients: A pilot randomized trial. Canadian Journal of Anesthesia [Internet]. 2012 Nov 30 [cited 2017 Aug 8];**59**(11):1032-1039. Available from: http://www.ncbi.nlm.nih.gov/pubmed/22932944

[61] Silverberg MJ, Li N, Acquah SO, Kory PD. Comparison of video laryngoscopy versus direct laryngoscopy during urgent endotracheal intubation: A randomized controlled trial. Critical Care Medicine [Internet]. 2014 Mar [cited 2017 Aug 8];**43**(3):717-718. Available from: http://www.ncbi.nlm.nih.gov/pubmed/25700064%5Cnhttp://www.ncbi.nlm.nih.gov/pubmed/25479112

[62] Janz DR, Semler MW, Lentz RJ, Matthews DT, Assad TR, Norman BC, et al. Randomized trial of video laryngoscopy for endotracheal intubation of critically ill adults. Critical Care Medicine [Internet]. 2016 Nov [cited 2017 Aug 8];**44**(11):1-8. Available from: http://www.ncbi.nlm.nih.gov/pubmed/27355526

[63] Lascarrou JB, Boisrame-Helms J, Bailly A, Le Thuaut A, Kamel T, Mercier E, et al. Video laryngoscopy vs direct laryngoscopy on successful first-pass orotracheal intubation among ICU patients a randomized clinical trial. JAMA [Internet]. 2017 Feb 7 [cited 2017 Aug 7];**317**(5):483-493. Available from: http://www.ncbi.nlm.nih.gov/pubmed/28118659

[64] De Jong A, Molinari N, Terzi N, Mongardon N, Arnal JM, Guitton C, et al. Early identification of patients at risk for difficult intubation in the intensive care unit: Development and validation of the MACOCHA score in a multicenter cohort study. American Journal

of Respiratory and Critical Care Medicine [Internet]. 2013 Apr 15 [cited 2017 Aug 7];**187**(8):832-839. Available from: http://www.ncbi.nlm.nih.gov/pubmed/23348979

[65]   Joshi R, Hypes CD, Greenberg J, Snyder L, Malo J, Bloom JW, et al. Difficult airway characteristics associated with first-attempt failure at intubation using video laryngoscopy in the intensive care unit. Annals of the American Thoracic Society [Internet]. 2017 Mar [cited 2017 Aug 2];**14**(3):368-375. Available from: http://www.atsjournals.org/doi/10.1513/AnnalsATS.201606-472OC

[66]   Su Y-C, Chen C-C, Lee Y-K, Lee J-Y, Lin KJ. Comparison of video laryngoscopes with direct laryngoscopy for tracheal intubation: A meta-analysis of randomised trials. European Journal of Anaesthesiology [Internet]. 2011 Nov [cited 2017 Aug 8];**28**(11):788-795. Available from: http://www.ncbi.nlm.nih.gov/pubmed/21897263

[67]   Michailidou M, O'Keeffe T, Mosier JM, Friese RS, Joseph B, Rhee P, et al. A comparison of video laryngoscopy to direct laryngoscopy for the emergency intubation of trauma patients. World Journal of Surgery [Internet]. 2015 Mar 28 [cited 2017 Aug 8];**39**(3):782-788. Available from: http://www.ncbi.nlm.nih.gov/pubmed/25348885

[68]   Sakles JC, Mosier J, Patanwala AE, Dicken J. Learning curves for direct laryngoscopy and GlideScope® video laryngoscopy in an emergency medicine residency. Western Journal of Emergency Medicine [Internet]. 2014 Nov 1 [cited 2017 Aug 7];**15**(7):930-937. Available from: http://www.ncbi.nlm.nih.gov/pubmed/25493156%5Cnhttp://www.pubmedcentral.nih.gov/articlerender.fcgi?artid=PMC4251257

[69]   Maharaj CH, Costello JF, Higgins BD, Harte BH, Laffey JG. Learning and performance of tracheal intubation by novice personnel: A comparison of the Airtraq® and Mancintosh laryngoscope. Anaesthesia [Internet]. 2006 Jul [cited 2017 Aug 7];**61**(7):671-677. Available from: http://www.ncbi.nlm.nih.gov/pubmed/16792613

[70]   Paolini JB, Donati F, Drolet P. Review article: Video-laryngoscopy: Another tool for difficult intubation or a new paradigm in airway management? Canadian Journal of Anesthesia. 2013;**60**(2):184-191

[71]   Narang AT, Oldeg PF, Medzon R, Mahmood AR, Spector JA, Robinett DA. Comparison of intubation success of video laryngoscopy versus direct laryngoscopy in the difficult airway using high-fidelity simulation. Simulation in Healthcare [Internet]. 2009 [cited 2017 Aug 8];**4**(3):160-165. Available from: http://www.ncbi.nlm.nih.gov/pubmed/19680083

[72]   Sakles JC, Mosier J, Chiu S, Cosentino M, Kalin L. A comparison of the C-MAC video laryngoscope to the macintosh direct laryngoscope for intubation in the emergency department. Annals of Emergency Medicine [Internet]. 2012 Dec [cited 2017 Aug 8];**60**(6):739-748. Available from: http://www.ncbi.nlm.nih.gov/pubmed/22560464

[73]   McElwain J, Malik MA, Harte BH, Flynn NM, Laffey JG. Comparison of the C-MAC® videolaryngoscope with the Macintosh, Glidescope®, and Airtraq® laryngoscopes in easy and difficult laryngoscopy scenarios in manikins. Anaesthesia [Internet]. 2010 May 19 [cited 2017 Aug 8];**65**(5):483-489. Available from: http://www.ncbi.nlm.nih.gov/pubmed/20337620

[74] Kim HJ, Chung SP, Park IC, Cho J, Lee HS, Park YS. Comparison of the GlideScope video laryngoscope and Macintosh laryngoscope in simulated tracheal intubation scenarios. Emergency Medicine Journal [Internet]. 2008 May 1 [cited 2017 Aug 8];**25**(5):279-282. Available from: http://www.ncbi.nlm.nih.gov/pubmed/18434462

[75] Lim Y, Yeo SW. A comparison of the GlideScope with the Macintosh laryngoscope for tracheal intubation in patients with simulated difficult airway. Anaesthesia & Intensive Care [Internet]. 2005 Apr [cited 2017 Aug 8];**33**(2):243-247. Available from: http://www.ncbi.nlm.nih.gov/pubmed/15960409

[76] Savoldelli GL, Schiffer E, Abegg C, Baeriswyl V, Clergue F, Waeber JL. Comparison of the Glidescope®, the McGrath®, the Airtraq® and the macintosh laryngoscopes in simulated difficult airways. Anaesthesia [Internet]. 2008 Dec [cited 2017 Aug 8];**63**(12):1358-1364. Available from: http://www.ncbi.nlm.nih.gov/pubmed/19032306

[77] Mosier JM, Stolz U, Chiu S, Sakles JC. Difficult airway management in the emergency department: GlideScope videolaryngoscopy compared to direct laryngoscopy. Journal of Emergency Medicine [Internet]. 2012 Jun [cited 2017 Aug 8];**42**(6):629-634. Available from: http://www.ncbi.nlm.nih.gov/pubmed/21911279

[78] Aziz MF, Healy D, Kheterpal S, Fu RF, Dillman D, Brambrink AM. Routine clinical practice effectiveness of the glidescope in difficult airway management. Anesthesiology [Internet]. 2011 Jan [cited 2017 Aug 8];**114**(1):34-41. Available from: http://www.ncbi.nlm.nih.gov/pubmed/21150569

[79] Park SO, Kim JW, Na JH, Lee KH, Lee KR, Hong DY, et al. Video laryngoscopy improves the first-attempt success in endotracheal intubation during cardiopulmonary resuscitation among novice physicians. Resuscitation [Internet]. 2015 Apr [cited 2017 Aug 8];**89**(C):188-194. Available from: http://www.ncbi.nlm.nih.gov/pubmed/25541427

[80] Lee DH, Han M, An JY, Jung JY, Koh Y, Lim CM, et al. Video laryngoscopy versus direct laryngoscopy for tracheal intubation during in-hospital cardiopulmonary resuscitation. Resuscitation [Internet]. 2015 Apr [cited 2017 Aug 8];**89**(C):195-199. Available from: http://www.ncbi.nlm.nih.gov/pubmed/25541431

[81] Ural K, Subaiya C, Taylor C, Ramadhyani U, Scuderi-Porter H, Nossaman BD. Analysis of orotracheal intubation techniques in the intensive care unit. Critical Care and Resuscitation [Internet]. 2011 Jun [cited 2017 Aug 8];**13**(2):89-96. Available from: http://www.ncbi.nlm.nih.gov/pubmed/21627576

[82] Noppens RR, Geimer S, Eisel N, David M, Piepho T. Endotracheal intubation using the C-MAC® video laryngoscope or the Macintosh laryngoscope: a prospective, comparative study in the ICU. Critical Care [Internet]. 2012 Jun 13 [cited 2017 Aug 8];**16**(3):R103. Available from: http://www.pubmedcentral.nih.gov/articlerender.fcgi?artid=3580658&tool=pmcentrez&rendertype=abstract

[83] Lakticova V, Koenig SJ, Narasimhan M, Mayo PH. Video laryngoscopy is associated with increased first pass success and decreased rate of esophageal intubations during

urgent endotracheal intubation in a medical intensive care unit when compared to direct laryngoscopy. Journal of Intensive Care Medicine [Internet]. 2015 Jan 13 [cited 2017 Aug 8];**30**(1):44-48. Available from: http://jic.sagepub.com/content/30/1/44.long

[84] Seupaul RA, Jones JH. Evidence-based emergency medicine. Does succinylcholine maximize intubating conditions better than rocuronium for rapid sequence intubation? Annals of Emergency Medicine [Internet]. 2011 Mar [cited 2017 Aug 8];**57**(3):301-302. Available from: http://linkinghub.elsevier.com/retrieve/pii/S0196064410012072

[85] Lysakowski C, Suppan L, Czarnetzki C, Tassonyi E, Tramèr MR. Impact of the intubation model on the efficacy of rocuronium during rapid sequence intubation: Systematic review of randomized trials. Acta Anaesthesiologica Scandinavica [Internet]. 2007 Aug [cited 2017 Aug 7];**51**(7):848-857. Available from: http://www.ncbi.nlm.nih.gov/pubmed/17635392

[86] Álvarez Gómez JA, Ariño Irujo JJ, Errando Oyonarte CL, Martínez Torrente F, Roigé i Solé J, Gilsanz Rodríguez F. Empleo clínico de bloqueantes neuromusculares y su reversión. Recomendaciones del grupo de expertos de la Sociedad Española de Anestesiología, Reanimación y Tratamiento del Dolor. Revista Española de Anestesiología y Reanimación [Internet]. 2009 Jan [cited 2017 Aug 8];**56**(10):616-627. Available from: http://linkinghub.elsevier.com/retrieve/pii/S0034935609704785

[87] Tran DTT, Newton EK, Mount VAH, Lee JS, Wells GA, Perry JJ. Rocuronium versus succinylcholine for rapid sequence induction intubation. In: The Cochrane Collaboration, editor. The Cochrane Database of Systematic Reviews [Internet]. Chichester, UK: John Wiley & Sons, Ltd; 2015 [cited 2017 Aug 6]. p. CD002788. Available from: http://doi.wiley.com/10.1002/14651858.CD002788.pub3

[88] Algie CM, Mahar RK, Tan HB, Wilson G, Mahar PD, Wasiak J. Effectiveness and risks of cricoid pressure during rapid sequence induction for endotracheal intubation. In: Wasiak J, editor. The Cochrane Database of Systematic Reviews [Internet]. Chichester, UK: John Wiley & Sons, Ltd; 2015 [cited 2017 Aug 7]. p. CD011656. Available from: http://www.ncbi.nlm.nih.gov/pubmed/26578526

[89] Schmidt UH, Kumwilaisak K, Bittner E, George E, Hess D. Effects of supervision by attending anesthesiologists on complications of emergency tracheal intubation. Anesthesiology [Internet]. 2008 Dec [cited 2017 Aug 7];**109**(6):973-977. Available from: papers3://publication/doi/10.1097/ALN.0b013e31818ddb90

[90] Dixon BJ, Dixon JB, Carden JR, Burn AJ, Schachter LM, Playfair JM, et al. Preoxygenation is more effective in the 25 degrees head-up position than in the supine position in severely obese patients: A randomized controlled study. Anesthesiology [Internet]. 2005 Jun [cited 2017 Aug 7];**102**(6):1110-1115; discussion 5A. Available from: http://www.ncbi.nlm.nih.gov/pubmed/15915022

[91] Ramkumar V, Umesh G, Ann Philip F. Preoxygenation with 20° head-up tilt provides longer duration of non-hypoxic apnea than conventional preoxygenation in non-obese healthy adults. Journal of Anesthesia [Internet]. 2011 Apr 4 [cited 2017 Aug 7];**25**(2):189-194. Available from: http://www.ncbi.nlm.nih.gov/pubmed/21293885

[92] Norris MC, Kirkland MR, Torjman MC, Goldberg ME. Denitrogenation in pregnancy. Canadian Journal of Anesthesia [Internet]. 1989 Sep [cited 2017 Aug 7];36(5):523-525. Available from: http://www.ncbi.nlm.nih.gov/pubmed/2791175

[93] Carmichael FJ, Cruise CJE. Preoxygenation—A study of denitrogenation.pdf. Obstetric Anesthesia Digest [Internet]. 1989 Mar [cited 2017 Aug 7];68(3):406-409. Available from: http://www.ncbi.nlm.nih.gov/pubmed/2493208

[94] Hubert S, Massa H, Ruggiu G, Raucoules-Aimé M. Preoxigenación en anestesia. EMC—Anestesia-Reanimación. 2009;35(3):1-6.

[95] Preoxygenation: Physiology and practice. Lancet [Internet]. 1992 Jan 4 [cited 2017 Aug 7]; 339(8784):31-32. Available from: http://www.ncbi.nlm.nih.gov/pubmed/1345958

[96] De Jong A, Futier E, Millot A, Coisel Y, Jung B, Chanques G, et al. How to preoxygenate in operative room: healthy subjects and situations "at risk." Annales Françaises D'anesthèsie et de Rèanimation [Internet]. 2014 Jul [cited 2017 Aug 7];33(7-8):457-461. Available from: http://www.ncbi.nlm.nih.gov/pubmed/25168301

[97] Mort TC. Preoxygenation in critically ill patients requiring emergency tracheal intubation. Critical Care Medicine [Internet]. 2005 Nov [cited 2017 Aug 7];33(11):2672-2675. Available from: http://www.ncbi.nlm.nih.gov/entrez/query.fcgi?cmd=Retrieve&db=PubMed&dopt=Citation&list_uids=16276196

[98] Baillard C, Fosse JP, Sebbane M, Chanques G, Vincent F, Courouble P, et al. Noninvasive ventilation improves preoxygenation before intubation of hypoxic patients. American Journal of Respiratory and Critical Care Medicine [Internet]. 2006 Jul 15 [cited 2017 Aug 7];174(2):171-177. Available from: http://www.ncbi.nlm.nih.gov/pubmed/16627862

[99] Findley LJ, Ries AL, Tisi GM, Wagner PD. Hypoxemia during apnea in normal subjects: Mechanisms and impact of lung volume. Journal of Applied Physiology [Internet]. 1983 Dec [cited 2017 Aug 7];55(6):1777-1783. Available from: http://www.ncbi.nlm.nih.gov/pubmed/6662768

[100] Barjaktarevic I, Berlin D. Bronchoscopic intubation during continuous nasal positive pressure ventilation in the treatment of hypoxemic respiratory failure. Journal of Intensive Care Medicine [Internet]. 2013 Mar 15 [cited 2017 Aug 7];30(3):161-166. Available from: http://www.ncbi.nlm.nih.gov/pubmed/24243561

[101] Ricard J-D. High flow nasal oxygen in acute respiratory failure. Minerva Anestesiologica [Internet]. 2012 Jul [cited 2017 Aug 8];78(7):836-841. Available from: http://www.ncbi.nlm.nih.gov/pubmed/22531566

[102] Vourc'h M, Asfar P, Volteau C, Bachoumas K, Clavieras N, Egreteau PY, et al. High-flow nasal cannula oxygen during endotracheal intubation in hypoxemic patients: A randomized controlled clinical trial. Intensive Care Medicine [Internet]. 2015 Sep [cited 2017 Aug 7];41(9):1538-1548. Available from: http://www.ncbi.nlm.nih.gov/pubmed/25869405

[103] Constantin J-M, Futier E, Cherprenet A-L, Chanques G, Guerin R, Cayot-Constantin S, et al. A recruitment maneuver increases oxygenation after intubation of hypoxemic intensive

care unit patients: a randomized controlled study. Critical Care [Internet]. 2010 [cited 2017 Aug 7];**14**(2):R76. Available from: http://www.ncbi.nlm.nih.gov/pubmed/20426859

[104] Futier E, Constantin J-M, Petit A, Jung B, Kwiatkowski F, Duclos M, et al. Positive end-expiratory pressure improves end-expiratory lung volume but not oxygenation after induction of anaesthesia. European Journal of Anaesthesiology [Internet]. 2010 Apr [cited 2017 Aug 7];**27**(6):508-513. Available from: http://www.ncbi.nlm.nih.gov/pubmed/20404729

[105] Haddad F, Hunt SA, Rosenthal DN, Murphy DJ. Right ventricular function in cardio-vascular disease, part I: Anatomy, physiology, aging, and functional assessment of the right ventricle. Circulation [Internet]. 2008 Mar 18 [cited 2017 Aug 7];**117**(11):1436-1448. Available from: http://www.ncbi.nlm.nih.gov/pubmed/18347220

[106] Dewhirst E, Frazier WJ, Leder M, Fraser DD, Tobias JD. Cardiac arrest following ket-amine administration for rapid sequence intubation. Journal of Intensive Care Medicine [Internet]. 2012 Nov 29 [cited 2017 Aug 7];**28**(6):375-379. Available from: http://www.ncbi.nlm.nih.gov/pubmed/22644454

[107] Martinez Hurtado E, Sanchez Merchante M. Commentary to "Hemodynamic response to endotracheal intubation using C-Trach assembly and direct laryngoscopy". Saudi Journal of Anaesthesia [serial online] 2016 [cited 2017 Nov 22];**10**:485-486. Available from: http://europepmc.org/abstract/med/27833506

[108] De Backer D, Biston P, Devriendt J, Madl C, Chochrad D, Aldecoa C, et al. Comparison of dopamine and norepinephrine in the treatment of shock. New England Journal of Medicine [Internet]. 2010 Mar 4 [cited 2017 Aug 7];**362**(9):779-789. Available from: http://www.ncbi.nlm.nih.gov/pubmed/20200382

[109] Ripollés-Melchor J, Casans-Francés R, Espinosa A, Abad-Gurumeta A, Feldheiser A, López-Timoneda F, et al. Goal directed hemodynamic therapy based in esophageal Doppler flow parameters: A systematic review, meta-analysis and trial sequential analysis. Revista Española de Anestesiología y Reanimación (English Ed). 2016 Aug-Sep;**63**(7):384-405. doi: 10.1016/j.redar.2015.07.009. Epub 2016 Feb 10

[110] Ripollés J, Espinosa A, Martínez-Hurtado E, Abad-Gurumeta A, Casans-Francés R, Fernández-Pérez C, et al. Intraoperative goal directed hemodynamic therapy in non-cardiac surgery: A systematic review and meta-analysis | Terapia hemodinâmica alvo-dirigida no intraoperatório de cirurgia não cardíaca: revisão sistemática e meta-análise. Brazilian Journal of Anesthesiology [Internet]. 2016 Sep-Oct;**66**(5):513-528. doi: 10.1016/j.bjane.2015.02.001. Epub 2015 Sep 14

[111] Monnet X, Letierce A, Hamzaoui O, Chemla D, Anguel N, Osman D, et al. Arterial pressure allows monitoring the changes in cardiac output induced by volume expan-sion but not by norepinephrine. Critical Care Med [Internet]. 2011 Jun [cited 2017 Aug 7];**39**(6):1394-1399. Available from: http://www.ncbi.nlm.nih.gov/pubmed/21336124

[112] Loubani OM, Green RS. A systematic review of extravasation and local tissue injury from administration of vasopressors through peripheral intravenous catheters and central

venous catheters. Journal of Critical Care [Internet]. 2015 Jun [cited 2017 Aug 7];**30**(3):653. e9-653.e17. Available from: http://www.ncbi.nlm.nih.gov/pubmed/25669592

[113] Krishnan S, Schmidt GA. Acute right ventricular dysfunction: Real-time management with echocardiography. Chest [Internet]. 2015 Mar [cited 2017 Aug 7];**147**(3):835-846. Available from: http://www.ncbi.nlm.nih.gov/pubmed/25732449

[114] Calvo-Vecino JM, Hernández EV, Rodríguez JMR, Segurola CL, Trapero CM, Quintas CN, et al. Vía Clínica de Recuperación Intensificada en Cirugía Abdominal (RICA). Instituto Aragonés de Ciencias de la Salud. 2014.

[115] Leeuwenburg T. Airway management of the critically ill patient: Modifications of traditional rapid sequence induction and intubation. Critical Care Horizons [Internet]. 2015;**1**(1):1-10. Available from: http://www.criticalcarehorizons.com/wp-content/uploads/2014/06/airway-management-critically.pdf

[116] Greyson CR. Ventrículo derecho y circulación pulmonar: Conceptos básicos. Revista Española de Cardiología [Internet]. 2010 [cited 2017 Aug 2];**63**(1):81-95. Available from: http://linkinghub.elsevier.com/retrieve/pii/S0300893210700129

[117] Lupi-Herrera E, Santos Martínez L-E, Figueroa Solano J, Sandoval Zárate J. [Homeometric autoregulation in the heart. The Anrep effect. Its possible role in increased right ventricular afterload pathophysiology]. Archivos de Cardiologia de Mexico [Internet]. [cited 2017 Aug 7];**77**(4):330-348. Available from: http://www.ncbi.nlm.nih.gov/pubmed/18361080

[118] Dalabih M, Rischard F, Mosier JM. What's new: The management of acute right ventricular decompensation of chronic pulmonary hypertension. Intensive Care Medicine [Internet]. 2014 Dec 3 [cited 2017 Aug 7];**40**(12):1930-1933. Available from: http://www.ncbi.nlm.nih.gov/pubmed/25183571

[119] Germann P, Braschi A, Della Rocca G, Dinh-Xuan AT, Falke K, Frostell C, et al. Inhaled nitric oxide therapy in adults: European expert recommendations. Intensive Care Medicine [Internet]. 2005 Aug 23 [cited 2017 Aug 7];**31**(8):1029-1041. Available from: http://www.ncbi.nlm.nih.gov/pubmed/15973521

[120] Howell JB, Permutt S, Proctor DF, Riley RL. Effect of inflation of the lung on different parts of pulmonary vascular bed. Journal of Applied Physiology [Internet]. 1961 Jan [cited 2017 Aug 7];**16**:71-76. Available from: http://www.ncbi.nlm.nih.gov/pubmed/13716268

[121] Jaber S, Jung B, Corne P, Sebbane M, Muller L, Chanques G, et al. An intervention to decrease complications related to endotracheal intubation in the intensive care unit: A prospective, multiple-center study. Intensive Care Medicine [Internet]. 2010 Feb 17 [cited 2017 Aug 7];**36**(2):248-255. Available from: http://www.ncbi.nlm.nih.gov/pubmed/19921148

[122] Langeron O, Amour J, Vivien B, Aubrun F. Clinical review: Management of difficult airways. Critical Care. 2006;**10**(6):243

[123] Mariscal Flores M, Martínez Hurtado E, Cuesta R, Jiménez MJ. ¿Existe un Gold Standard en el manejo de la VAD? Revisión 2015. Revista Electrónica de AnestesiaR [Internet]. 2016;8(2):384. Available from: http://anestesiar.org/rear/volumen-viii-2016/ numero-02/659-existe-un-gold-standard-en-el-manejo-de-la-via-aerea-dificil-revision-2015

[124] Serocki G, Bein B, Scholz J, Dörges V. Management of the predicted difficult airway: A comparison of conventional blade laryngoscopy with video-assisted blade laryngoscopy and the GlideScope. European Journal of Anaesthesiology. 2010;27(1):24-30.

[125] Mariscal Flores M, Martinez Hurtado E. Platform CIP, editor. Actualizaciones en VAD: Puesta al dia—2014-2015 [Internet]. 1st ed. AnestesiaR; 2014. 274 p. Available from: https://www.amazon.es/Actualizaciones-Via-Aerea-Dificil-Puesta/dp/1503008037·

[126] Palencia-Herrejon E, Borrallo-Perez JM, Pardo-Rey C. Intubation of the critical patient. Medicina Intensiva. 2008;32(1):3-11

[127] Fenwick R. Rapid sequence induction in urgent care settings. Emergency Nurse [Internet]. 2014 Mar 5 [cited 2017 Aug 7];21(10):16-24. Available from: http://www.ncbi.nlm.nih.gov/ pubmed/24597816

[128] Cormack RS, Lehane J. Difficult tracheal intubation in obstetrics. Anaesthesia. 1984; 39(11):1105-1111

[129] Pearce A. Evaluation of the airway and preparation for difficulty. Best Practice & Research Clinical Anaesthesiology [Internet]. 2005 Dec [cited 2017 Aug 7];19(4):559-579. Available from: http://www.ncbi.nlm.nih.gov/pubmed/16408534

[130] Brichant JF. [The Helsinki declaration on patient safety in anaesthesiology]. Acta Anaesthesiologica Belgica [Internet]. 2010 Jul [cited 2017 Aug 7];61(2):49. Available from: http://content.wkhealth.com/linkback/openurl?sid=WKPTLP:landingpage&an=0000 3643-201007000-00003

[131] Valero R, Sabaté S, Borràs R, Áñez C, Bermejo S, González-Carrasco FJ, Andreu E, Villalonga R, López A, Villalonga A, Massó E. Secció de Via Aèria de la Societat Catalana d'Anestesiologia, Reanimació i Terapèutica del Dolor. Recomendaciones sobre seguridad del paciente quirúrgico. Protocolo de manejo de la vía aérea difícil. Implicación de la Declaración de Helsinki. Difficult airway management protocol. Involvement of the Declaration of Helsinki. Revista Española de Anestesiología y Reanimación [Internet]. 2013;60(Supl 1):34-45. DOI: 10.1016/S0034-9356(13)70008-2 (https://goo.gl/7zpeFn)

[132] Woodall N, Frerk C, Cook TM. Can we make airway management (even) safer?—Lessons from national audit. Anaesthesia [Internet]. 2011 Dec [cited 2017 Aug 7];66(Suppl. 2):27-33. Available from: http://www.ncbi.nlm.nih.gov/pubmed/22074076

[133] Metzner J, Posner KL, Lam MS, Domino KB. Closed claims' analysis. Best Practice & Research Clinical Anaesthesiology. 2011;25(2):263-276

[134] Lewis SR, Butler AR, Parker J, Cook TM, Smith AF. Videolaryngoscopy versus direct laryngoscopy for adult patients requiring tracheal intubation. In: Lewis SR, editor. Cochrane Database of Systematic Reviews [Internet]. Chichester, UK: John Wiley & Sons, Ltd; 2016 [cited 2017 Aug 8]. p. CD011136. Available from: http://www.ncbi.nlm. nih.gov/pubmed/27844477

[135] Cook TM, Astin JP, Kelly FE. Airway Management in ICU: Three Years on from NAP4. ICU. 2014;**142**(2). Matrix (https://goo.gl/a8wKhi)

[136] Wetsch WA, Carlitscheck M, Spelten O, Teschendorf P, Hellmich M, Genzwurker H V, et al. Success rates and endotracheal tube insertion times of experienced emergency physicians using five video laryngoscopes: A randomised trial in a simulated trapped car accident victim. European Journal of Anaesthesiology [Internet]. 2011;**28**(12):849-858. Available from: http://www.ncbi.nlm.nih.gov/pubmed/21986981

[137] Martínez-Hurtado E, Lucena de Pablo E, Sanchez Merchante M, De Luis Cabezón N. Videolaryngoscopy data record. A reality that is possible. In: Conference: World Airway Management Meeting Website—WAMM2015, At Dublin [Internet]. 2015. Available from: https://www.researchgate.net/publication/283720966_Videolaryngoscopy_ Data_Record_A_Reality_That_Is_Possible

Abdominal Compartment Syndrome: What Is New?

Abdulgafoor M. Tharayil, Adel Ganaw,
Syed Abdulrahman, Zia M. Awan and
Sujith M. Prabhakaran

Abstract

Intra-abdominal hypertension (IAH) and abdominal compartment syndrome (ACS) are continuation of the same pathological and physiological processes that are largely unrecognized in critical patients. From an era of indistinct definitions and recommendations, this condition has been studied extensively and experts have come forward with clear definitions and recommendations for management. IAH is graded in four grades and ACS is IAH above 20 cm H_2O with new organ dysfunction. IAH/ACS can present as acute, hyperacute, or chronic and aetiologically can be classified into primary, secondary and tertiary. It affects various body systems including respiratory, cardiovascular, central nervous, gastrointestinal, renal and hepatic systems adversely and results in deleterious consequences. Management of IAH/ACS is based on the evacuation of intra-luminal and extra-luminal contents, improving the abdominal wall compliance. There are various surgical techniques recommended for preventing the development of IAH/ACS and mitigating the negative consequences. New medical therapies such as octreotide, tissue plasminogen activator, melatonin and vitamin C are being investigated and non-pharmacological methods such as continuous negative abdominal pressure (CNAP) have been introduced recently but are still experimental and not recommended for routine use.

Keywords: intra-abdominal hypertension (IAH), abdominal compartment syndrome (ACS), open abdomen

1. Introduction

Intra-abdominal hypertension (IAH) and abdominal compartment syndrome (ACS) are largely unrecognized conditions but prevalent in ICU patients. It is a continuum of varying degree of increase in intra-abdominal pressure (IAP) ranging from IAH to ACS. Most studies evaluating the incidence of ACS have been performed in trauma patients, with estimates of incidence varying considerably. While the largest study [1] ($n = 706$) reported an incidence of ACS of 1%, two smaller though observational studies [2, 3] ($n = 128$ and 188) reported a higher incidence of ACS of 9–14%. The incidence of intra-abdominal hypertension (IAH) is not well reported in the literature. The wide variation in the reported incidence may be attributed to differences in diagnostic criteria employed in studies.

2. Definitions

There was an era of indistinct and variable definitions of IAH/ACS with variable methods of measurement of intra-abdominal pressure (IAP) until the World Society of Abdominal Compartment Syndrome (WSACS) was formed and they formulated definitions, standardized measurement methodology and provided management guidelines.

Intra-abdominal pressure: Intra-abdominal pressure (IAP) is the steady state pressure concealed within the abdominal cavity (**Figure 1**) [4]. An IAP of 5–7 mmHg is considered normal for most critically ill patients. IAP is directly related to body mass index (BMI) [5].

Abdominal perfusion pressure: Abdominal perfusion pressure (APP) is calculated by subtracting IAP from the mean arterial pressure (MAP): APP = MAP – IAP. Elevated intra-abdominal pressure reduces blood flow to the abdominal viscera. A target APP of at least 60 mmHg is correlated with improved survival among patients with IAH and ACS [6].

Intra-abdominal hypertension: Intra-abdominal hypertension (IAH) is defined as a sustained intra-abdominal pressure ≥12 mmHg (**Figure 1**) [7, 8]. This value was established arbitrarily. Intra-abdominal pressure can be further graded as follows:

Grade I = IAP 12–15 mmHg
Grade II = IAP 16–20 mmHg
Grade III = IAP 21–25 mmHg
Grade IV = IAP > 25 mm Hg

Hyper-acute IAH refers to elevation of the intra-abdominal pressure lasting only seconds due to any strenuous physical activity, sneezing, coughing, laughing, straining, or defecation, etc.

Acute IAH refers to elevation of the intra-abdominal pressure that develops over hours, which occurs usually due to surgical causes. Sub-acute IAH refers to elevation of the intra-abdominal pressure that develops over days usually due to medical conditions.

Chronic IAH refers to elevation of intra-abdominal pressure that develops over months (pregnancy) or years (morbid obesity)]. Chronic elevation of IAP usually does not result in ACS unless it is superimposed on acute or sub-acute IAH.

Abdominal compartment syndrome: ACS is defined as a sustained intra-abdominal pressure >20 mmHg (with or without APP <60 mmHg) that is associated with new organ dysfunction [4, 7, 8].

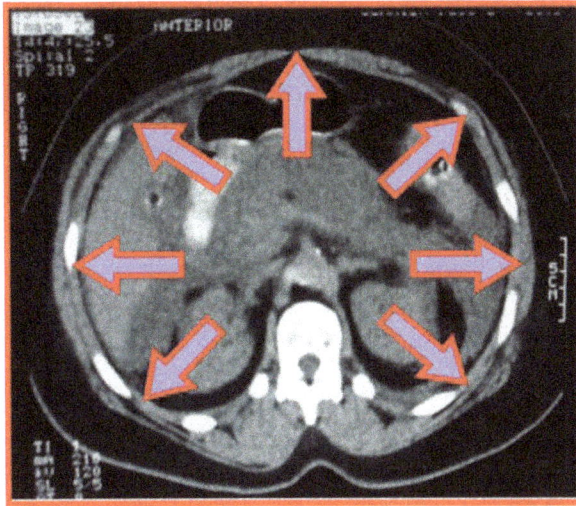

Figure 1. Intra-abdominal pressure (from: https://www.slideshare.net/drabdulgafoormt/intraabdominal-hypertension).

ACS can be classified as primary and secondary.

Primary ACS is due to injury or disease in the abdominopelvic region. This could be intra-luminal or extra-luminal causes. Extra-luminal causes could be any pathology causing intra-abdominal collections outside the bowel lumens e.g. abdominal trauma, hemoperitoneum and pancreatitis. IAH/ACS can also develop due to intra-luminal pathology like intestinal obstruction, gastroparesis, pseudocolonic obstruction and pseudomembranous colitis (**Figure 2**), etc.

Secondary ACS refers to conditions that do not originate in the abdomen or pelvis (e.g. fluid resuscitation, sepsis, and burns).

Recurrent ACS defines a condition in which ACS develops again following previous surgical or medical treatment of primary or secondary ACS [9].

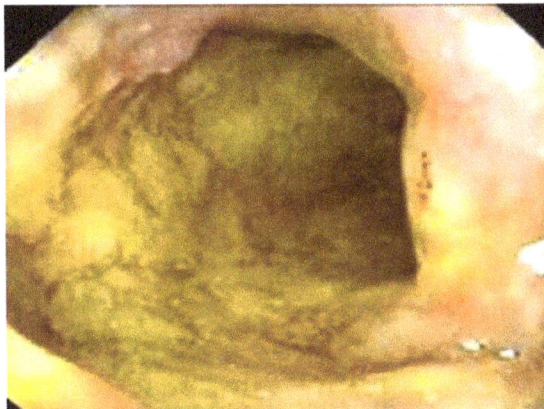

Figure 2. Pseudomembranous colitis due to clostridium difficile causing ACS [49].

3. Physiological consequences of IAH/ACS

ACS is not just an abdominal condition but rather a systemic problem that has tremendous impact on all organ systems including, but not limited to, cardiovascular system, respiratory system, central nervous system, renal system and hepatobiliary system.

Cardiovascular system: IAH/ACS results in cephalad movement of diaphragm that in turn can cause depression of ventricular compliance and contractility [10]. Another impact of IAH is reduced venous return from lower extremities that results in reduced preload and stagnation of blood in lower extremities causing deep vein thrombosis (DVT) [11].

Pulmonary system: Increased peak inspiratory and mean airway pressures induced by high IAP in mechanically ventilated patients can cause alveolar barotrauma. Associated with reduced chest wall compliance and reduced spontaneous tidal volumes, this cause arterial hypoxemia and hypercarbia. Pulmonary infection is also more common among patients with IAH [12]. According to animal studies, these effects are mediated through compression of the lung leading to atelectasis, oedema, increased intrapulmonary shunt fraction, decreased gas transfer and increased alveolar dead space [13].

Renal system: Kidney is affected by IAH/ACS by two ways: by direct compression of renal vein and by increased renal vasoconstriction caused by renin angiotensin induced by the decrease in preload.

The renal filtration gradient (FG) can be considered as the net force across the glomerulus. It is the gradient between the glomerular filtration pressure (GFP) and the proximal tubular pressure (PTP). In the presence of IAH, PTP is same as IAP. GFP is equivalent to the mean arterial pressure (MAP), and thus GFP can be estimated as MAP minus twice the IAP. Thus, the impact of IAP on the renal function and urine production is much greater than that caused by changes in MAP. So oliguria manifest is one of the first visible signs of IAH [14].

Filtration gradient: glomerular filtration pressure – proximal tubular pressure.

$$
\begin{aligned}
FG \ &= GFP - PTP \\
&= (MAP - IAP) - PTP \\
&= (MAP - IAP) - IAP \\
&= MAP - 2 \times IAP
\end{aligned}
\tag{1}
$$

Hence, when IAP is doubled, filtration gradient will be decreased by four-folds. Oliguria generally develops at an intra-abdominal pressure of approximately 15 mmHg, while anuria usually develops at an intra-abdominal pressure of approximately 30 mmHg [15]. Because of impairment in renal perfusion, the urine sodium and chloride concentrations are usually decreased. Along with increased plasma renin activity, aldosterone concentration and antidiuretic hormone concentration are also increased to more than twice their baseline levels, which has tremendous impact on the renal function [16].

Gastrointestinal system: The gut is very sensitive to increase in IAP as the primary organ is exposed to high IAP, which can occur at IAP as low as 10 mmHg [17]. At 20 mmHg of IAP mucosal perfusion pressure of the gut is decreased [18] and at 40 mmHg celiac and superior mesenteric blood flow are reduced [19]. IAH also impairs venous flow from the intestine by compressing intestinal veins and causes intestinal oedema. This increases intra-abdominal pressure further, as a vicious cycle [20]. This leads to worsened hypo perfusion, bowel ischemia, decreased intra-mucosal pH and lactic acidosis [21]. Hypoperfusion of the gut may result in loss of the mucosal barrier, leading to bacterial translocation, sepsis and multiple system organ failure. Bacterial translocation has been shown to occur at IAP of only 10 mmHg in the presence of haemorrhage [22].

Hepatic: Liver is affected by IAH by reducing its ability to clear lactate even with adequate cardiac output and blood pressure and this can occur with IAP as low as 10 mmHg [23].

Central nervous system: The effect of IAH on intracranial pressure (ICP) range from transient increases during the short-lived elevation of intra-abdominal pressure that occurs with coughing, defecating or emesis to sustained elevation during persistent elevation of IAH. This can lead to a critical decrease in cerebral perfusion pressure (CPP) [24]. Decompressive laparotomy was found to decrease ICP drastically in a case of ACS as reported by Bloomfield et al. [25].

4. Diagnosis

Physical examination was found to be neither sensitive nor specific for the diagnosis of IAH/ACS with a sensitivity of 56%, specificity of 87%, positive predictive value of 35%, negative predictive value of 94% and accuracy of 84% [26]. Imaging studies such as chest X-ray, ultrasound abdomen and CT scan are not useful to diagnose IAH/ACS efficiently but can give some clue to the possibility, such as elevated diaphragm, basal atelectasis, inferior venae caval compression, tense infiltration of the retro peritoneum that is out of proportion to peritoneal disease, massive abdominal distension, direct renal compression or displacement, bowel wall thickening or bilateral inguinal herniation [27].

Various techniques have been described for IAP measurement using intra-vesical, intra-gastric or inferior venae caval catheters. WSACS has standardized intra-vesical (urinary bladder) pressure measurement as the gold standard for measurement of IAH/ACS [28]. This was done through puncturing the aspiration port of Folley's catheter or attaching a three-way stopcock and connecting it to a manometer, but nowadays a closed system has been developed which avoids the puncturing and ensures sterility (**Figure 3**). The pressure is measured at end-expiration in the supine position after ensuring that abdominal muscle contractions are absent. The transducer should be zeroed at the level of the mid-axillary line. WSACS has also standardized the amount of saline to be instilled as up to 25 ml. However, as a downside, the bladder pressure may be inaccurate in the presence of intra-peritoneal adhesions, pelvic hematomas, pelvic fractures, abdominal packs or a neurogenic bladder [29].

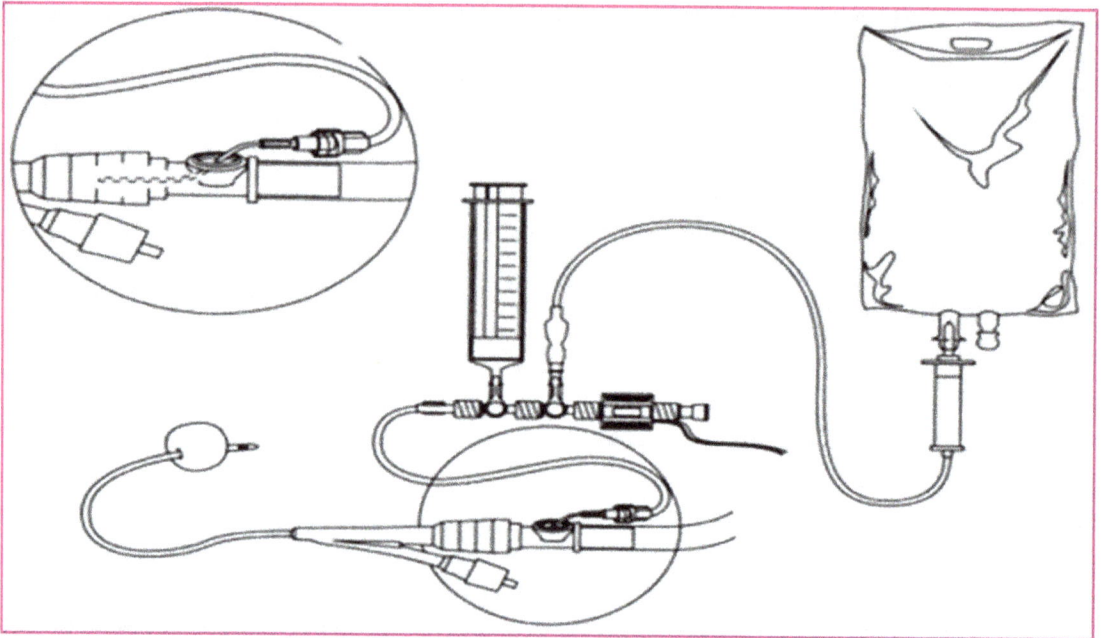

Figure 3. Closed system for intra-abdominal pressure monitoring (adapted from: Roberto et al. [50]).

5. Management of IAH/ACS

Surgical decompression is the definitive management of IAH/ACS but supportive medical therapy should be attempted before resorting to this. WSACS has provided algorithm for management of IAH/ACS (**Algorithms 1** and **2**). Nowadays, the trend is more towards less invasive management such as abdominal wall escharotomy in burns [30] or percutaneous drainage of intra-abdominal collections [31].

Principles of supportive care are [32] as follows:

1. *Evacuate intra-luminal contents*: nasogastric and rectal drainage.

2. *Drain extra-luminal collections*: evacuate hemoperitoneum, ascites, intra-abdominal abscess and retroperitoneal hematoma.

3. *Improve abdominal wall compliance*: supine position, adequate analgesia, sedation and sometimes muscle paralysis.

Many of IAH/ACS patients will need ventilatory support and should have a lung protective strategy like low tidal volume, pressure limitation, permissive hypercapnea, use of positive end expiratory pressure (PEEP) and use of muscle relaxants in indicated patients.

Aggressive fluid resuscitation is one of the risk factors for the development of ACS. As these patients are haemodynamically unstable initially, they receive large amounts of crystalloids with resultant bowel oedema and development or aggravation of ACS. Liberal use of colloids

WSACS — The Abdominal Compartment Society

IAH/ACS Management Algorithm

Intra-Abdominal Hypertension (IAH)

Patient has IAH (IAP ≥ 12 mmHg) — NO

Initiate treatment to reduce IAP
Avoid excessive fluid resuscitation
Optimize organ perfusion
(GRADE 1C)

IAP > 20 mmHg with new organ failure? — NO — Monitor IAP with serial measurements at least every 4 hours while patient is critically ill (GRADE 1C)

IAP < 12 mmHg consistently?

YES

Patient has ACS

YES — IAH has resolved Discontinue IAP measurements and monitor patient for clinical deterioration

Medical treatment options to reduce IAP
1. Improve abdominal wall compliance
   Sedation & analgesia
   Neuromuscular blockade
   Avoid head of bed > 30 degrees
2. Evacuate intra-luminal contents
   Nasogastric decompression
   Rectal decompression
   Gastro-/colo-prokinetic agents
3. Evacuate abdominal fluid collections
   Paracentesis
   Percutaneous drainage
4. Correct positive fluid balance
   Avoid excessive fluid resuscitation
   Diuretics
   Colloids / hypertonic fluids
   Hemodialysis / ultrafiltration
5. Organ Support
   Optimize ventilation, alveolar recruitment
   Use transmural (tm) airway pressures
   $Pplat_{tm}$ = Plat - 0.5 * IAP
   Consider using volumetric preload indices
   If using PAOP/CVP, use transmural pressures
   $PAOP_{tm}$ = PAOP - 0.5 * IAP
   CVP_{tm} = CVP - 0.5 * IAP

Abdominal Compartment Syndrome (ACS)

IDENTIFY AND TREAT UNDERLYING ETIOLOGY FOR PATIENT'S ACS

Does patient have Primary ACS? — NO — Patient has Secondary or Recurrent ACS

YES

Perform / revise abdominal decompression with temporary abdominal closure as needed to reduce IAP (GRADE 2D) — YES — Is IAP > 20 mmHg with progressive organ failure?

NO

Continue medical treatment options to reduce IAP (GRADE 1C)

Measure IAP at least every 4 hours while patient is critically ill (GRADE 1C)

Perform balanced resuscitation of patient preload, contractility, and afterload using crystalloid / colloid / vasoactive medications AVOID EXCESSIVE FLUID RESUSCITATION (GRADE 2D)

Is IAP > 20 mmHg with organ failure? — NO — Is IAP < 12 mmHg consistently? — YES — IAH has resolved Decrease frequency of IAP measurements and observe patient for deterioration

Definitions
IAH - intra-abdominal hypertension
ACS - abdominal compartment syndrome
IAP - intra-abdominal pressure
APP - abdominal perfusion pressure (MAP-IAP)
Primary ACS - A condition associated with injury or disease in the abdomino-pelvic region that frequently requires early surgical or interventional radiological intervention
Secondary ACS - ACS due to conditions that do not originate from the abdomino-pelvic region
Recurrent ACS - The condition in which ACS redevelops following previous surgical or medical treatment of primary or secondary ACS

Adapted from Intensive Care Med 2013 7:1190-1206
© 2014 World Society of the Abdominal Compartment Syndrome. All rights reserved.

World Society of the Abdominal Compartment Syndrome (WSACS)
Tel: +32 929 802 36
Website: http://www.wsacs.org
e-mail: info@wsacs.org

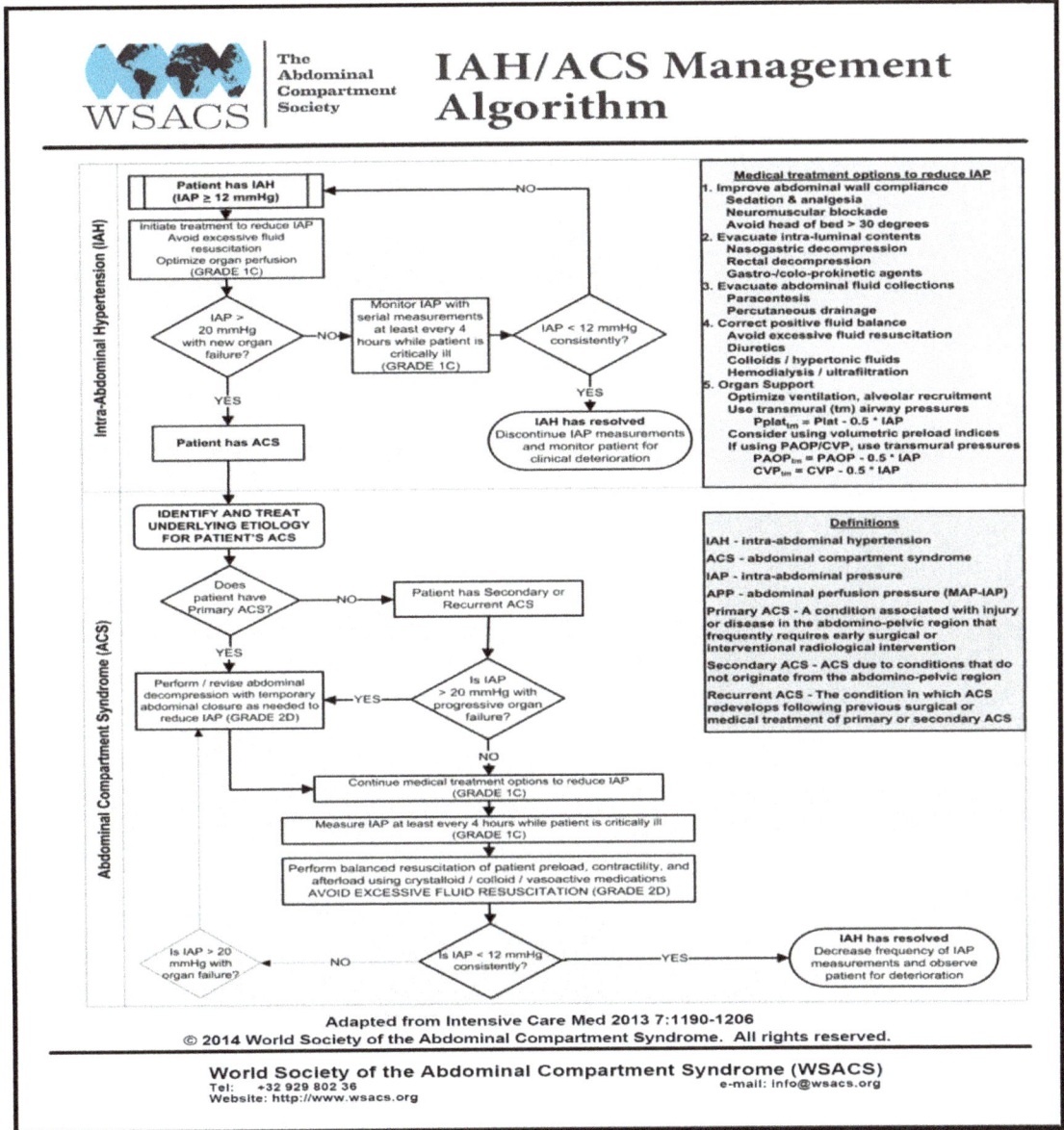

Algorithm 1. Management of IAH/ACS by WSACS: Adapted from World Society of the Abdominal Compartment Syndrome (WSACS) website: http://www.wsacs.org.

has not yet proved to prevent this. But on the other side optimum fluid resuscitation can prevent some negative aspects of ACS such as reduced cardiac output, renal blood flow, urine output and visceral perfusion.

Decompressive laparotomy is the definitive treatment for ACS. Many surgeons resort to decompression when the IAP is above 25, but a lower threshold would be better in terms of organ saving. An approach based on abdominal perfusion pressure (APP) rather than IAP would be more logical, and a threshold APP of 50 mmHg was found to correlate with mortality [33].

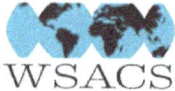

The Abdominal Compartment Society

WSACS

IAH/ACS Medical Management Algorithm

- The choice (and success) of the medical management strategies listed below is strongly related to both the etiology of the patient's IAH / ACS and the patient's clinical situation. The appropriateness of each intervention should always be considered prior to implementing these interventions in any individual patient.
- The interventions should be applied in a stepwise fashion until the patient's intra-abdominal pressure (IAP) decreases. If there is no response to a particular intervention, therapy should be escalated to the next step in the algorithm.

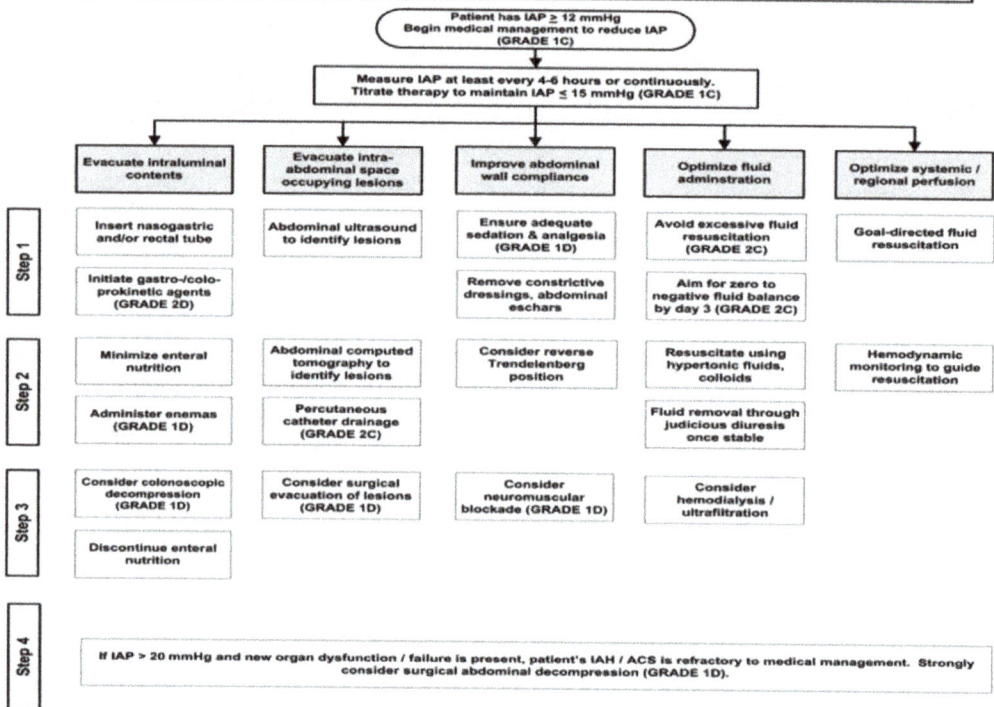

Patient has IAP ≥ 12 mmHg
Begin medical management to reduce IAP
(GRADE 1C)

Measure IAP at least every 4-6 hours or continuously.
Titrate therapy to maintain IAP ≤ 15 mmHg (GRADE 1C)

Evacuate intraluminal contents	Evacuate intra-abdominal space occupying lesions	Improve abdominal wall compliance	Optimize fluid administration	Optimize systemic / regional perfusion
Step 1 Insert nasogastric and/or rectal tube	Abdominal ultrasound to identify lesions	Ensure adequate sedation & analgesia (GRADE 1D)	Avoid excessive fluid resuscitation (GRADE 2C)	Goal-directed fluid resuscitation
Initiate gastro-/colo-prokinetic agents (GRADE 2D)		Remove constrictive dressings, abdominal eschars	Aim for zero to negative fluid balance by day 3 (GRADE 2C)	
Step 2 Minimize enteral nutrition	Abdominal computed tomography to identify lesions	Consider reverse Trendelenberg position	Resuscitate using hypertonic fluids, colloids	Hemodynamic monitoring to guide resuscitation
Administer enemas (GRADE 1D)	Percutaneous catheter drainage (GRADE 2C)		Fluid removal through judicious diuresis once stable	
Step 3 Consider colonoscopic decompression (GRADE 1D)	Consider surgical evacuation of lesions (GRADE 1D)	Consider neuromuscular blockade (GRADE 1D)	Consider hemodialysis / ultrafiltration	
Discontinue enteral nutrition				

Step 4 If IAP > 20 mmHg and new organ dysfunction / failure is present, patient's IAH / ACS is refractory to medical management. Strongly consider surgical abdominal decompression (GRADE 1D).

Adapted from Intensive Care Med 2013 7:1190-1206
© 2014 World Society of the Abdominal Compartment Syndrome. All rights reserved.

World Society of the Abdominal Compartment Syndrome (WSACS)
Tel: +32 929 802 36   e-mail: info@wsacs.org
Website: http://www.wsacs.org

Algorithm 2. Medical management of IAH/ACS by WSACS: Adapted from World Society of the Abdominal Compartment Syndrome (WSACS) website: http://www.wsacs.org.

An open abdomen approach after decompression with temporary closure methods is commonly used by most surgeons to prevent recurrent ACS.

There are different methods for managing open abdomen (OA). Abdomen can be closed with temporary abdominal closure using various techniques, which should be later followed by interval abdominal closure, by bringing the edges of the abdominal fascia together primarily (primary closure) if possible technically. If technically not feasible, OA can be closed either using a functional closure or simple coverage [34]. Negative pressure techniques like vacuum-assisted closure (VAC) (**Figure 4**), patch technique (e.g. Whittmann patch, polytetrafluoroethylene patch),

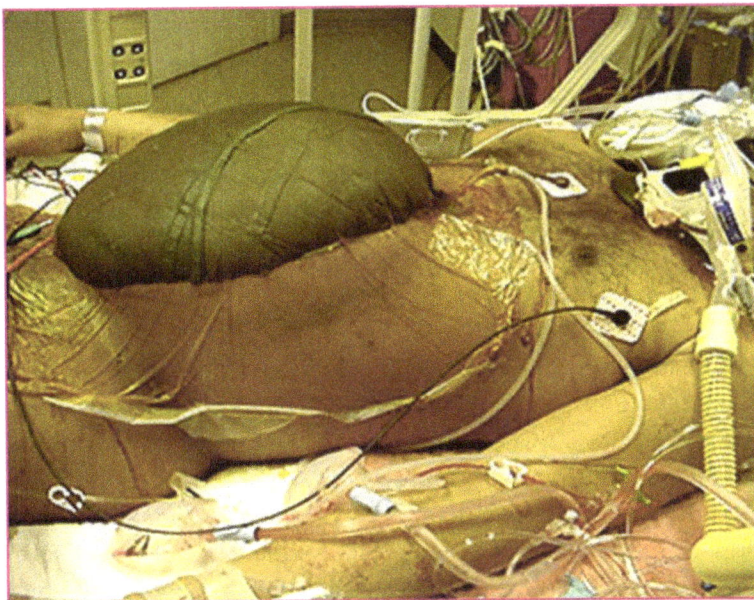

Figure 4. Vacuum-assisted closure (from: https://www.slideshare.net/drabdulgafoormt/intraabdominal-hypertension).

silo technique (e.g. Bagota bag) (**Figure 5**) and skin-only technique using towel clips are some methods used in the management of open abdomen. Each technique has its own advantages and disadvantages and description of that is beyond the scope of this chapter.

Closure of abdomen after the ACS also utilizes different methods such as STAR (staged abdominal repair), component separation and planned ventral hernia. An international consensus conference on open abdomen in Trauma [35] concluded that open abdomen (OA) in trauma is advisable at the end of damage-control laparotomy, especially in the presence of swelling of viscera, for a second look if there are vascular injuries or gross contamination of

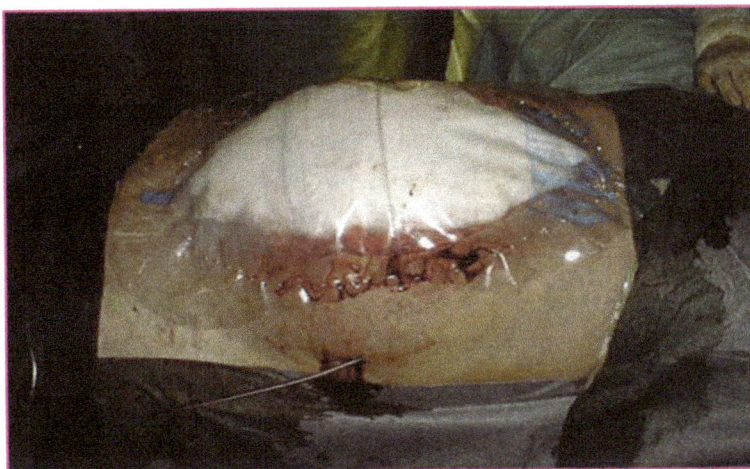

Figure 5. Bagota bag closure (from Huang et al. [51]).

the peritoneal cavity, or if there is loss of abdominal wall, and in cases of failure of medical treatment of abdominal compartment syndrome, but early closure is mandatory to prevent complications such as fistulae formation and frozen abdomen. A review by Sugrue M, opined that the key to optimizing outcome in ACS is early abdominal closure within 7 days because failure to do so increases morbidity, mortality and fistulae formation [36].

6. Recent insights

In a recent experimental study, Leng et al. [37] indicated that mitochondrial Ca^{2+}uptake 1 (MICU1)-related oxidation/antioxidation disequilibrium is strongly involved in IAH-induced damage to intestinal barriers. MICU1-targeted treatment may hold promise for preventing the progression of IAH to gut-derived sepsis. Earlier in 2014, an animal study led by the same author found that acute exposure to slightly elevated IAP may result in adverse effects on intestinal permeability and the pro-oxidant-antioxidant balance and so monitoring IAP is very important in critical patients [38]. In another experiment in rats by Liu et al. [39], Melanocortin 4 (MC4 receptor) agonist counteracts the intestinal inflammatory response, ameliorating intestinal injury in experimental secondary IAH by MC4 receptor-triggered activation of the cholinergic anti-inflammatory pathway. This may represent a promising strategy for the treatment of IAH in the future.

A systematic review and individual patient data meta-analysis on intra-abdominal hypertension in critically ill patients: the wake-up project (World initiative on Abdominal Hypertension Epidemiology, a Unifying Project) [40] in 2014 looking at the outcome and mortality in IAH/ACS found that the only independent predictors for IAH were SOFA score and fluid balance on the day of admission. 513 patients out of 2707 patients (30.8%) died in ICU. The independent predictors for intensive care mortality were SAPS II score, IAH, SOFA score and admission category. This review showed that IAH is an independent predictor for mortality and is frequently present in critically ill patients more than anticipated.

New medical treatment options that are still experimental include tissue plasminogen activator (tPa), theophylline and octreotide. tPa was evaluated for retroperitoneal hematoma by Horer et al. [41]. They analysed 13 patients who developed ACS with multiple organ failure in the ICU. The mean IAP was 23.5 mmHg before decompression (range 12–35), and when tPA was given, IAP dropped to a mean of 16 mmHg (range 10–28.5) after 24 h of administration. Drainage of hematoma after tPa increased to 1520 mL (range 170–2900) from 370 mL (range 5–1000). This also coincided with improvement in urinary output and haemodynamics.

Bodnar et al. [42] found a positive correlation between IAH and increased levels of serum adenosine and interleukin10 concentrations in 45 surgical patients with IAP >12 mmHg. Based on these findings, they conducted another study [43] comparing standard medical treatment in patients with IAH versus standard medical treatment and theophylline infusions twice daily. Mortality in theophylline group was 0% when compared to standard group (55%). Theophylline improved renal function, splanchnic perfusion, and cardiac contractility possibly by counteracting adenosine binding to adenosine receptors. The authors postulated that by decreasing circulating adenosine concentrations, theophylline infusion improves IAH-related mortality in surgical patients

Octreotide, a synthetic somatostatin analogue, by decreasing myeloperoxidase (MPO) activity and malondialdehyde levels and thereby increasing levels of glutathione if given before decompression of IAP has been shown to improve the reperfusion-induced oxidative damage in rats with ACS [44]. This translates to that octreotide might have a therapeutic role as an agent limiting reperfusion injury among patients with IAH and ACS.

Free radical scavengers such as melatonin and vitamin C (ascorbic acid) were also tried in the medical management of IAH/ACS and found useful in animal studies [45]. Vitamin C was found to reduce resuscitation fluid requirements significantly thereby preventing secondary ACS and IAH in burns [46].

Another nonsurgical technique being investigated is continuous negative extra-abdominal pressure (CNAP). Bloomfield et al. [47] demonstrated a significant reduction in IAP when continuous negative pressure was applied by vacuum via a large poncho into which the entire animal was placed. There was a mean reduction in IAP from 30.7 ± 1.3 to 18.2 ± 1.3 mmHg. Apart from IAP, central venous pressure (CVP), inferior venae caval (IVC) pressure, intra cranial pressure (ICP), pulmonary artery occlusion pressure (PAOP) and peak airway pressure were also reduced. This was also evaluated in a human study by Sugerman et al. [48], which proved the above benefits although some patients expressed discomfort in lower chest and pelvic area. All the novel medical options for management of IAH/ACS apart from standard medical management-like evacuation of intra and extra luminal contents, improvement of abdominal wall compliance, are still in experimental stage and not recommended for routine use.

7. Conclusion

IAH/ACS is not a problem limited to the abdomen but rather a systemic problem affecting various body systems adversely with deleterious consequences. Addressing this important pathology in a timely manner is crucial for the better outcome of critically ill patients. Mainstay of the management in IAH/ACS is still surgical decompression but medical options are equally important interventions. Novel therapies in medical options are being explored and needs further validation to be recommended in routine management of patients with intra-abdominal hypertension and abdominal compartment syndrome.

Author details

Abdulgafoor M. Tharayil*, Adel Ganaw, Syed Abdulrahman, Zia M. Awan and Sujith M. Prabhakaran

*Address all correspondence to: atharayil@hamad.qa

Department of Anaesthesia, Hamad Medical Corporation, Doha, Qatar

References

[1] Hong JJ, Cohn SM, Perez JM, Dolich MO, Brown M, McKenney MG. Prospective study of the incidence and outcome of intra-abdominal hypertension and the abdominal compartment syndrome. British Journal of Surgery. 2002;**89**(5):591

[2] Balogh Z, McKinley BA, Holcomb JB, Miller CC, Cocanour CS, Kozar RA, Valdivia A, Ware DN, Moore FA. Both primary and secondary abdominal compartment syndrome can be predicted early and are harbingers of multiple organ failure. Journal of Trauma. 2003;**54**(5):848

[3] Balogh Z, McKinley BA, Cocanour CS, Kozar RA, Holcomb JB, Ware DN, Moore FA. Secondary abdominal compartment syndrome is an elusive early complication of traumatic shock resuscitation. American Journal of Surgery. 2002;**184**(6):538

[4] Malbrain ML, Cheatham ML, Kirkpatrick A, Sugrue M, Parr M, De Waele J, Balogh Z, Leppäniemi A, Olvera C, Ivatury R, D'Amours S, Wendon J, Hillman K, Johansson K, Kolkman K, Wilmer A. Results from the International Conference of experts on intra-abdominal hypertension and abdominal compartment syndrome. I. Definitions. Intensive Care Medicine. 2006;**32**(11):1722

[5] Sanchez NC, Tenofsky PL, Dort JM, Shen LY, Helmer SD, Smith RS. What is normal intra-abdominal pressure? American Surgeon. 2001;**67**(3):243

[6] Schein M, Ivatury R. Intra-abdominal hypertension and the abdominal compartment syndrome. British Journal of Surgery. 1998;**85**(8):1027.

[7] Vidal MG, Ruiz Weisser J, Gonzalez F, Toro MA, Loudet C, Balasini C, Canales H, Reina R, Estenssoro E. Incidence and clinical effects of intra-abdominal hypertension in critically ill patients. Critical Care Medicine. 2008;**36**(6):1823

[8] http://www.wsacs.org/consensus_summary.php [Accessed on October 11, 2011].

[9] Van Mook WN, Huslewe-Evers RP, Ramsay G. Abdominal compartment syndrome. Lancet. 2002;**360**(9344):1502

[10] Cullen DJ, Coyle JP, Teplick R, Long MC. Cardiovascular, pulmonary, and renal effects of massively increased intra-abdominal pressure in critically ill patients. Critical Care Medicine. 1989;**17**(2):118.

[11] Barnes GE, Laine GA, Giam PY, Smith EE, Granger HJ. Cardiovascular responses to elevation of intra-abdominal hydrostatic pressure. American Journal of Physiology. 1985;**248**(2 Pt 2):R208.

[12] Aprahamian C, Wittmann DH, Bergstein JM, Quebbeman EJ. Temporary abdominal closure (TAC) for planned relaparotomy (etappenlavage) in trauma. Journal of Trauma. 1990;**30**(6):719

[13] Quintel M, Pelosi P, Caironi P, Meinhardt JP, Luecke T, Herrmann P, Taccone P, Rylander C, Valenza F, Carlesso E, Gattinoni L. An increase of abdominal pressure increases

pulmonary edema in oleic acid-induced lung injury. American Journal of Respiratory Critical Care Medicine. 2004;**169**(4):534

[14] Papavramidis TS, Marinis AD, Pliakos I, Kesisoglou I, Papavramidou N. Abdominal compartment syndrome – Intra-abdominal hypertension: Defining, diagnosing, and managing. Journal of Emergencies, Trauma and Shock. 2011;**4**(2):279-291

[15] Richards WO, Scovill W, Shin B, Reed W. Acute renal failure associated with increased intra-abdominal pressure. Annals of Surgery. 1983;**197**(2):183-187.

[16] Le Roith D, Bark H, Nyska M, Glick SM. The effect of abdominal pressure on plasma antidiuretic hormone levels in the dog. Journal of Surgical Research. 1982;**32**(1):65

[17] Friedlander MH, Simon RJ, Ivatury R, DiRaimo R, Machiedo GW. Effect of hemorrhage on superior mesenteric artery flow during increased intra-abdominal pressures. Journal of Trauma. 1998;**45**(3):433

[18] Chang MC, Cheatham ML, Nelson LD, Rutherford EJ, Morris JA Jr. Gastric tonometry supplements information provided by systemic indicators of oxygen transport. Journal of Trauma. 1994;**37**(3):488

[19] Caldwell CB, Ricotta JJ. Changes in visceral blood flow with elevated intraabdominal pressure. Journal of Surgical Research. 1987;**43**(1):14

[20] Mark G. Abdominal compartment syndrome in adults. In: Hilary S, Eileen MB, editors. Up to Date. Waltham, MA. [Accessed on March 4, 2017]

[21] Diebel LN, Wilson RF, Dulchavsky SA, Saxe J. Effect of increased intra-abdominal pressure on hepatic arterial, portal venous, and hepatic microcirculatory blood flow. Journal of Trauma. 1992;**33**(2):279

[22] Gargiulo NJ 3rd, Simon RJ, Leon W, Machiedo GW. Hemorrhage exacerbates bacterial translocation at low levels of intra-abdominal pressure. Archives of Surgery. 1998;**133**(12):1351

[23] Luca A, Cirera I, García-Pagán JC, Feu F, Pizcueta P, Bosch J, Rodés J. Hemodynamic effects of acute changes in intra-abdominal pressure in patients with cirrhosis. Gastroenterology. 1993;**104**(1):222

[24] Citerio G, Vascotto E, Villa F, Celotti S, Pesenti A. Induced abdominal compartment syndrome increases intracranial pressure in neurotrauma patients: A prospective study. Critical Care Medicine. 2001;**29**(7):1466.

[25] Bloomfield GL, Dalton JM, Sugerman HJ, Ridings PC, DeMaria EJ, Bullock R. Treatment of increasing intracranial pressure secondary to the acute abdominal compartment syndrome in a patient with combined abdominal and head trauma. Journal of Trauma. 1995;**39**(6):1168

[26] Kirkpatrick AW, Brenneman FD, McLean RF, Rapanos T, Boulanger BR. Is clinical examination an accurate indicator of raised intra-abdominal pressure in critically injured patients? Canadian Journal of Surgery. 2000;**43**(3):207

[27] Pickhardt PJ, Shimony JS, Heiken JP, Buchman TG, Fisher AJ. The abdominal compartment syndrome: CT findings. American Journal of Roentgenology. 1999;**173**(3):575

[28] Kirkpatrick AW, Roberts DJ, De Waele J, Jaeschke R, Malbrain ML, De Keulenaer B, Duchesne J, Bjorck M, Leppaniemi A, Ejike JC, Sugrue M, Cheatham M, Ivatury R, Ball CG, Reintam Blaser A, Regli A, Balogh ZJ, D'Amours S, Debergh D, Kaplan M, Kimball E, Olvera C. Pediatric guidelines sub-committee for the world society of the abdominal compartment syndrome. Intra-abdominal hypertension and the abdominal compartment syndrome: Updated consensus definitions and clinical practice guidelines from the World Society of the Abdominal Compartment Syndrome. Intensive Care Medicine. 2013;**39**(7):1190-1206. Epub 2013 May 15.

[29] Malbrain ML. Different techniques to measure intra-abdominal pressure (IAP): Time for a critical re-appraisal. Intensive Care Medicine. 2004;**30**(3):357

[30] Hobson KG, Young KM, Ciraulo A, Palmieri TL, Greenhalgh DG. Release of abdominal compartment syndrome improves survival in patients with burn injury. Journal of Trauma. 2002;**53**(6):1129

[31] Cheatham ML, Safcsak K. Percutaneous catheter decompression in the treatment of elevated intraabdominal pressure. Chest. 2011;**140**(6):1428

[32] Cheatham ML. Nonoperative management of intraabdominal hypertension and abdominal compartment syndrome. World Journal of Surgery. 2009;**33**(6):1116-1122

[33] Cheatham ML, White MW, Sagraves SG, Johnson JL, Block EF. Abdominal perfusion pressure: A superior parameter in the assessment of intra-abdominal hypertension. Journal of Trauma. 2000;**49**(4):621

[34] Neils M, Babak S. In: Eileen M, Katthryn AC, editor. Up to Date. Waltham, MA. [Accessed on March 4, 2017]

[35] Chiara O, Cimbanassi S, Biffl W, Leppaniemi A, Henry S, Scalea, Thomas M, et al. Journal of Trauma and Acute Care Surgery. 2016;**80**(1):173-183

[36] Sugrue M. Abdominal compartment syndrome and the open abdomen: any unresolved issues? Current Opinion in Critical Care. 2017;**23**(1):73-78

[37] Leng Y, Ge Q, Zhao Z, Wang K, Yao G. MICU1 may be a promising intervention target for gut-derived sepsis induced by intra-abdominal hypertension. Cell Death Discovery. 2016;**2**:16080.

[38] Yuxin L,Kuo Z, Jie F, Min Y, Qinggang G, Li C, Lu Z, Gaiqi Y. Effect of acute, slightly increased intra-abdominal pressure on intestinal permeability and oxidative stress in a rat model. PLoS One. 2014;9(10) e109350.

[39] Liu D, Zhang HG, Chang MT, Li Y, Zhang LY. Melanocortin-4 receptor agonists alleviate intestinal dysfunction in secondary intra-abdominal hypertension rat model. Journal of Surgical Research. 2015;**195**(1):263-270

[40] Malbrain ML, Chiumello D, Cesana BM, Reintam Blaser A, Starkopf J, Sugrue M, Pelosi P. A systematic review and individual patient data meta-analysis on intra-abdominal hypertension in critically ill patients: The wake-up project. World initiative on Abdominal Hypertension Epidemiology, a Unifying Project (WAKE-Up!). Minerva Anaesthesiology. 2014;**80**(3):293-306.

[41] Horer T, Skoog P, Pirouzram A, Larzon T. Tissue plasminogen activator-assisted hematoma evacuation to relieve abdominal compartment syndrome after endovascular repair of ruptured abdominal aortic aneurysm. Journal of Endovascular Therapy. 2012;**19**:144–148

[42] Bodnar Z, Keresztes T, Kovacs I, Hajdu Z, Boissonneault GA, Sipka S. Increased serum adenosine and interleukin 10 levels as new laboratory markers of increased intra-abdominal pressure. Langenbecks Archives of Surgery. 2010;**395**:969–972

[43] Bodnar Z, Szentkereszty Z, Hajdu Z, Boissonneault GA, Sipka S. Beneficial effects of theophylline infusions in surgical patients with intra-abdominal hypertension. Langenbecks Archives of Surgery. 2011;**396**:793–800

[44] De Keulenaer B, Regli A, De laet I, Roberts DJ, Malbrain MLNG. What's new in medical management strategies for raised intra-abdominal pressure: Evacuating intra-abdominal contents, improving abdominal wall compliance, pharmacotherapy, and continuous negative extra-abdominal pressure. Anaesthesiology Intensive Therapy. 2015;**47**(1):54-62.

[45] Sener G, Kacmaz A, User Y, Ozkan S, Tilki M, Yegen BC. Melatonin ameliorates oxidative organ damage induced by acute intra-abdominal compartment syndrome in rats. Journal of Pineal Research. 2003;**35**:163–168

[46] Kremer T, Harenberg P, Hernekamp F et al. High-dose vitamin C treatment reduces capillary leakage after burn plasma transfer in rats. Journal of Burn Care Research. 2010;**31**:470–479

[47] Bloomfield G, Saggi B, Blocher C, Sugerman H. Physiologic effects of externally applied continuous negative abdominal pressure for intra-abdominal hypertension. Journal of Trauma. 1999;**46**:1009–1014

[48] Sugerman HJ, Felton IW, 3rd, Sismanis A, et al. Continuous negative abdominal pressure device to treat pseudotumor cerebri. International Journal of Obesity and Related Metabolic Disorders. 2001;**25**: 486

[49] Nissar Shaikh, et al. A rare and unsuspected complication of Clostridium difficile infection. Intensive Care Medicine. 2008;**34**:963-966

[50] Roberto, et al. Procedures for monitoring intra-abdominal pressure. Review of Medical Sciences. 2007 Jan-Mar;**11**(1) Pinar del Río

[51] Huang Q, Li J, Lau W-Y. Techniques for abdominal wall closure after damage control laparotomy: From temporary abdominal closure to early/delayed fascial closure—A review. Gastroenterology Research and Practice. 2016;2016:15. Article ID 2073260. DOI: http://dx.doi.org/10.1155/2016/2073260

Permissions

The contributors of this book come from diverse backgrounds, making this book a truly international effort. This book will bring forth new frontiers with its revolutionizing research information and detailed analysis of the nascent developments around the world.

We would like to thank all the contributing authors for lending their expertise to make the book truly unique. They have played a crucial role in the development of this book. Without their invaluable contributions this book wouldn't have been possible. They have made vital efforts to compile up to date information on the varied aspects of this subject to make this book a valuable addition to the collection of many professionals and students.

This book was conceptualized with the vision of imparting up-to-date information and advanced data in this field. To ensure the same, a matchless editorial board was set up. Every individual on the board went through rigorous rounds of assessment to prove their worth. After which they invested a large part of their time researching and compiling the most relevant data for our readers.

The editorial board has been involved in producing this book since its inception. They have spent rigorous hours researching and exploring the diverse topics which have resulted in the successful publishing of this book. They have passed on their knowledge of decades through this book. To expedite this challenging task, the publisher supported the team at every step. A small team of assistant editors was also appointed to further simplify the editing procedure and attain best results for the readers.

Apart from the editorial board, the designing team has also invested a significant amount of their time in understanding the subject and creating the most relevant covers. They scrutinized every image to scout for the most suitable representation of the subject and create an appropriate cover for the book.

The publishing team has been an ardent support to the editorial, designing and production team. Their endless efforts to recruit the best for this project, has resulted in the accomplishment of this book. They are a veteran in the field of academics and their pool of knowledge is as vast as their experience in printing. Their expertise and guidance has proved useful at every step. Their uncompromising quality standards have made this book an exceptional effort. Their encouragement from time to time has been an inspiration for everyone.

The publisher and the editorial board hope that this book will prove to be a valuable piece of knowledge for researchers, students, practitioners and scholars across the globe.

List of Contributors

Miguel Ángel García García, Alfonso Martínez Cornejo and David Arizo León
Intensive Care Unit, Hospital de Sagunto, Valencia, Spain

María Ángeles Rosero Arenas
Primary Care, Cheste, Valencia, Spain

Adel E. Ahmed Ganaw, Abdulgafoor M. Tharayil, Ali O. Mohamed Bel Khair, Saher Tahseen, Jazib Hassan, Mohammad Faisal Abdullah Malmstrom and Sohel Mohamed Gamal Ahmed
Department of Anesthesiology, ICU and Perioperative Medicine, Hamad Medical Corporation, Doha, Qatar

Nandita Mehta and Sayyidah Aasima tu Nisa Qazi
Department of Anaesthesia and Critical Care, Acharya Shri Chander College of Medical Sciences and Hospital, Jammu, India

Arshad Chanda
Hamad General Hospital, Doha, State of Qatar

Jae H. Kim and Nikolai Shalygin
University of California San Diego and Rady Children's Hospital of San Diego, San Diego, California, USA

Azif Safarulla
Augusta University, Augusta, Georgia, USA

Melek Nihal Esin
Public Health Nursing Department, Florence Nightingale Nursing Faculty, Istanbul University, Istanbul, Turkey

Duygu Sezgin
Department of Nursing & Midwifery, Education & Health Sciences Faculty, University of Limerick, Limerick, Ireland

Eugenio Martinez Hurtado and Javier Ripolles Melchor
Department of Anaesthesia, Intensive Care Medicine and Pain Medicine, Hospital Universitario Infanta Leonor, Madrid, España

Miriam Sanchez Merchante
Department of Anaesthesia, Intensive Care Medicine and Pain Medicine, Hospital Universitario Fundación Alcorcón, Madrid, España

Sonia Martin Ventura and Maria Luisa Mariscal Flores
Department of Anaesthesia, Intensive Care Medicine and Pain Medicine, Hospital Universitario de Getafe, Madrid, España

Abdulgafoor M. Tharayil, Adel Ganaw, Syed Abdulrahman, Zia M. Awan and Sujith M. Prabhakaran
Department of Anaesthesia, Hamad Medical Corporation, Doha, Qatar

Index

A

Abdominal Compartment Syndrome, 72, 173-174, 179-180, 182-187

Acinetobacter Baumannii, 3, 9, 12

Acute Pancreatitis, 72-93

Airway Management, 127-128, 130, 132-133, 135, 139-140, 152, 154, 156-160, 162-163, 165-166, 170-172

Albumin, 24, 38, 44, 84

Alcohol Abuse, 27-28, 88

Anaesthesiologist, 51

Analgesia, 48, 67-68, 72, 88, 159-161, 178

Anastomotic Structure, 25

Aneurysm Morphology, 28

Aneurysmal Subarachnoid Hemorrhage, 24, 30, 33, 37, 49-50

Antibiotic Resistance, 1-3, 6-8, 10, 22-23

Antimicrobial, 7, 12, 23

Antithrombotic Therapy, 27

B

Balthazar Score, 72

C

Cardiac Complication, 24

Cardiomyopathy, 40, 51-59, 62-71

Cellular Ischemic Tolerance, 34

Central Venous Pressure, 42, 56-57, 62, 69, 183

Cerebral Blood Arteries, 34

Cerebral Edema, 28, 36, 44, 95

Cerebral Vasospasm, 31, 34-36, 38, 40, 43-44, 49

Cerebrospinal Fluid, 24, 28, 35, 48

Chronic Obstructive Pulmonary Disease, 3

Circle of Willis, 25

Clazosentan, 37

Colonization, 1-2, 4-5, 8-10, 13-14, 16, 21-22

D

Diabetes Mellitus, 3, 53, 92, 116

E

Echocardiography, 40, 55, 58-60, 63-64, 66-67, 69-70, 94, 97-98, 105-106, 170

Endothelin, 35, 37

Enterococcus Faecium, 3

Extraglottic Device, 135, 154-155

F

Fasudil, 36

G

Glasgow Score, 72

H

Hepatic, 96, 107, 173, 177, 185

Hospital Flora, 4

Hydrocephalus, 28, 33, 38-39, 48

Hyponatremia, 24, 39, 41-45, 50

I

Inferior Venae Caval, 177, 183

Inflammation, 27, 73, 75, 78, 81, 88, 115

Inflammatory Condition, 72

Intensive Care Unit, 1-2, 22-24, 43, 68, 105, 108-110, 114-115, 117-118, 122-124, 127, 159, 161-162, 164-167, 170

Intra-abdominal Hypertension, 87, 173-174, 182-187

Intracranial Aneurysm, 29, 33, 47

Intravascular Shear Stress, 28

Ischemia, 33-35, 37, 39, 43, 45, 49, 150, 177

K

Klebsiella Pneumoniae, 3-4

L

Laryngoscopy, 68, 127, 129, 133-136, 138-143, 145-146, 154, 157, 159, 161-167, 169, 171-172

Lumbar Puncture, 29, 49, 103, 108

M

Moyamoya Disease, 26

Multiorgan Failure, 72, 89

Multiresistant Bacteria, 1-2

Myeloperoxidase, 183

N

Necrotizing Enterocolitis, 94, 101, 107-108

Neurological Deficit, 30-31, 34, 36-38
Nimodipine, 35-36
Nosocomial Infection, 12

O
Occupational Health, 109, 112-113, 116-120, 122-123
Octreotide, 173, 182-183
Oropharynx, 4-6

P
Papaverine, 37
Pneumothorax, 94, 99, 106
Pseudocolonic Obstruction, 175
Pseudomonas Aeruginosa, 3, 12

S
Severe Acute Pancreatitis, 72-73, 76, 84-86, 88, 90-91
Staphylococcus Aureus, 3

Subarachnoid Hemorrhage, 24, 26, 29-30, 32-33, 37-38, 40, 45, 47-50
Subarachnoid Space, 26, 28-29
Systolic Blood Pressure, 33, 36, 151

T
Tracheal Intubation, 127, 131-135, 156-158, 160-161, 165-168, 171-172
Tracheostomy, 132

V
Vancomycin, 3-4, 8
Vasospasm, 24, 28, 31-40, 43-45, 47-49
Ventriculostomy, 33
Videolaryngoscope, 128, 141-142, 145-147, 163-165

X
Xanthochromia, 29

www.ingramcontent.com/pod-product-compliance
Lightning Source LLC
Chambersburg PA
CBHW062004190326

41458CB00009B/2966